Spared
A Memoir of Risk and Resolve

Lori Jones

SPARED
A Memoir of Risk and Resolve

This book is a memoir, based on true events. It reflects the author's present recollections of experiences over time. Some names and characteristics have been changed, some events have been compressed, and some dialogue has been recreated.

ISBN: 9798990798403

ACKNOWLEDGEMENTS

The Things We've Handed Down
Words and Music by Marc Cohn
Copyright © 1993 Sony Music Publishing (US) LLC
All Rights Administered by Sony Music Publishing (US) LLC, 424 Church Street, Suite 1200, Nashville, TN 37219
International Copyright Secured All Rights Reserved
Reprinted by Permission of Hal Leonard LLC

Cover Art by Alynn Olson
Author Photo Credits: Zaelynn Photography LLC
https://zaelynnphotographywi.com

Thank you to my family for being vulnerable and supporting this book.

DEDICATION

For Chris,
who was willing to take the risk.

You may not always be so grateful
For the way that you were made
Some feature of your father's
That you'd gladly sell or trade
And one day you may look at us
And say that you were cursed.

But over time that line has been
Extremely well rehearsed
By our fathers, and their fathers
In some old and distant town
From places no one here remembers
Come the things we've handed down.

"The Things We've Handed Down"

-Marc Cohn

CHAPTER 1
Polarity

Grandpa was an S.O.B. I knew this because Dad said so. I didn't know what an S.O.B. was at the time, but I knew it must be something bad, because of the way he said it and because of how Mom looked at him when he said it, a look that warned, "not in front of the children."

One of my earliest memories of my dad interacting with his own father conjures drowsy warmth conflicting with cold ankles, the winter day that Grandpa paid a visit to our house, unannounced.

In the mornings when I was not yet old enough for school, I would creep out to the kitchen in my nightgown and perch on the edge of the baseboard radiator. This was the best position from which to sit quietly and wait for either Mom or Dad to emerge from their bedroom or more likely, my sister to wake up and join me, her being tall enough to reach the cereal box and pour the milk.

The slim ledge of metal venting ran the length of our kitchen. When I sat on it and remained patiently, it gave off the most wonderful heat which crawled right up your back and under your neck. Then warm air blew out of the side slats, hitting your legs.

I was sitting on the radiator, feeling my stomach grumble, but basking in the toasted heat when the knock came. My insides did a lurch. People at the door were always a cause for alarm, especially if they were unexpected. I was beginning to grasp the concept, even at an early age, that visitors were never welcome in our home.

The rapping sounded again, louder, and more insistent. The knocker had come all the way up, climbed the green wooden steps outside, and then continued through the screen door and up more steps of the inside porch, which we called "The Green" because of its green carpet. He banged on the wooden door.

"What in the hell?" my father muttered, exiting their dark bedroom, and hurrying unsteadily through the kitchen, undressed and half-asleep, to peek through our peep hole.

We had a unique peep hole, not the dime-sized metal circle like I saw on the TV shows, where people lived in apartment buildings, but a small crack in the bottom corner of the frosted plexiglass. Earlier that year, Dad had glued the plastic sheeting over our window for what he called privacy. When the plexiglass chipped as he was bending it in, he said he had done it that way on purpose.

When it cracked, I had been watching him work, and I worried that there would be an angry storm, but he paused, took a deep breath, and craned his neck down.

"See, if you tilt your head just so, you can peek right through here and check who's out there before you answer." He explained, "Pretty ingenious of your 'Old Man,' huh?"

He meant smart, but I wasn't so sure, since we were never allowed to answer the door anyway, no matter who it was, but I had nodded in zealous agreement at the time.

When Dad saw through the opening that it was Grandpa, he swore a few choice words and turned the other direction. My stomach twisted in knots, as I thought he was going to leave Grandpa standing on the porch, but, eventually, he returned with, of all things, the shaggy bathroom rug wrapped around his naked waist.

Dad was not pleased about this company, and I could feel the vibration of his anger as clearly as the radiator heat wafting through my pajamas. He cracked the door, and the freezing air of the porch hit my bare ankles. It felt like ice and even more so because of how warm I was everywhere else. I wanted to curl my legs up under me, but I wouldn't have been able to balance that way on the ledge, so I resigned myself to my bipolar state.

Grandpa cautiously stepped a few feet into the kitchen.

He was wearing a hat with a cement company logo on it, navy canvas coveralls, and leather work boots. He smelled of gasoline, machine grease, and hard labor. He removed his hat and held it awkwardly in his hands.

My grandpa could fix anything. He ran his own excavating company, and when he wasn't operating huge Caterpillars to move mountains of soil, Grandpa was in his garage, tinkering on old cars and machine parts. I spent hours at Grandpa and Grandma's house, keeping him company in the garage, twirling on a stool and watching him work with his tools.

He would always pause and let me turn the final crank of the press or pound the last whack of a nail, claiming I would make a mighty fine mechanic someday with that grip or that aim. A part of me knew he was only joking, but the other part felt proud.

Then Grandma would call us for dinner from the house. Before heading in, you had to clean up, it was just like playing with my toys. Each tool had a home on the garage wall, with a nail hook and an outline of its shape in Sanford permanent black marker. We made a game of finding the right tool to fill each shadow.

Then before going in to eat, we would wash the grease from our hands at the outdoor sink, using gritty Lava soap which scraped you up, but in a good way. No matter how hard Grandpa scrubbed, he always had remnants of black grease under his fingernails and in the cracks of his knuckles. I guessed when you put that much hard work into a day, it didn't come back out of you very easily.

Grandpa surveyed the scene and took in our dark little kitchen, Dad sporting disheveled bed hair, gripping the bathmat toga around him, and me, a small shadow of a girl willing herself to disappear. My grandpa could fix anything, but I didn't think he could fix this.

"Hello there, Sweetheart." He shifted nervously, rotating the hat, and smiled at me. I smiled back but didn't dare speak or move from my spot on the ledge.

I do not remember what they talked about. The conversation went quietly for a few minutes. It seemed Grandpa was trying to reason with my dad about something. Eventually their voices grew louder and escalated until Dad, securing the rug in place with one hand, pointed with the other and told Grandpa to leave.

"Son, be reasonable." Grandpa said, and then something under his breath like, "Just look at yourself."

But Dad persisted, holding his arm straight out, trembling finger aimed at the door. With wild eyes he ordered, "This is my home. Get out."

And Grandpa did.

I was sorry for Grandpa and somewhat embarrassed for him as well, a man in charge who nobody ever told what to do.

He put his Ready-Mix trucker hat back on his head, nodded at me and tried to smile like this had been a normal visit, but the twinkle usually found in his eyes wasn't there. He turned and left defeated, descending the steps, and shaking his head in wonder at this episode.

Dad slammed the door and locked it again. "That takes care of that," he pronounced, tightening the rug purposefully around his waist.

The other side of me felt kind of proud of my dad. He was tough and told that guy off. He had defended his domain. I sensed he had somehow protected us, but from what? The frigid air swirled with the slam and then diminished, as with mixed feelings I relaxed back into the comfort of the radiator, but although the warmth returned to my legs and feet, the schism in my heart could not be resolved.

CHAPTER 2
Career Liar

Years later I learned that blow up was Dad's last chance of being gainfully employed by what he called "The Man," which was the establishment, and "The Old Man," who was his father.

Dad had lasted approximately three days with Grandpa as the boss of him before telling Grandpa what he could do with his job. Prior to that my father held various positions, none of which lasted long. Career opportunities were limited in our small town in southern Wisconsin, especially if you didn't finish high school, and you had a short fuse to boot.

Despite his tough exterior, Dad was artistic. We had paintings hanging in our apartment that he had done before I was born, but it seemed an abandoned hobby that wouldn't have paid the bills anyway. Dad ran reels at the local movie theatre, punched a clock at a factory, and then stirred chocolate as a bakery chef. Before trying to work for Grandpa, Dad's most recent and longest stint was as the custodian for a school district just across the border in Illinois.

Dad repeatedly claimed that he couldn't read and couldn't write, but I had proof otherwise. One afternoon he returned from his shift at the school and slipped a small mustard yellow cardboard square from his pocket, handing it to me with a smile. As I turned it over and examined it, he said he'd "made it in Art class." Dad had pressed a tiny dandelion blossom flat and modge-podged it with some sort of acrylic to its frame. On the back he had inscribed in misspelled cursive, *"your sweet as a rose & I love you, Dad - '74."* I clung to this two-inch symbol of his love like a talisman and later slipped it into my keepsake box.

Although the janitorial job was stable, with two little girls and an added commute, it made sense for Mom to keep her steady position at the data center and for Dad to stay home with us. This arrangement didn't feel too off to me until I had other families to compare it to by way of the public school system.

In Kindergarten 1975 teachers still did a round table, all us kids sitting pretzel-legged on the carpet, sharing, "What does your Daddy do?" when called on. Ellen's dad was a businessman who traveled, her mother owned a shop downtown. He was her stepdad, and she called him by his first name, which made her seem exotic and more grown up to me. Kathy's parents both worked at a travel agency. Bruce's father was a doctor, and his mom was a homemaker. I became increasingly uneasy, as none of the answers around the circle involved a dad who stayed home. Even Carla, who said she didn't have a dad, which prompted Mrs. H. to move it along, seemed better than my situation. My dad stayed home and did what?

When it was my turn, I announced loudly, "My dad has a hurt back, and so he stays home and takes care of me and my sister. My mom is a keypuncher at the data center, and she works with big computers, like this big." I stretched out my arms as far as they would go.

And so began my future as a career-liar. I would spend the next 25 years defending Dad's slow but steady decline, which brought increasing physical symptoms and outrageous psychological behaviors. I would alternate between putting together the pieces of the Huntington's disease puzzle and burying my head in the sand of denial.

CHAPTER 3
Anomalies

In the 1970's, the proportion of fathers who stayed home with the children while their wives worked was 1% of the population, as estimated by the Pew Research Center. Our family hunkered well below that percentage, into the decimals, the odds of a stay-at-home dad also coming down with Huntington's disease.

Huntington's disease (HD) is a progressive and degenerative hereditary illness, affecting movement and cognition. HD results in a loss of coordination, involuntary movements, and psychiatric symptoms. The early indicators of HD can be behavioral and include everything from a lack of emotion and recognizing the needs of others, to aggression, excitability, and depression.

According to the Huntington's Disease Society of America (HDSA) there are currently approximately 41,000

Americans who are symptomatic and more than 200,000 living at risk of inheriting the disease.

In our family's arrangement, Mom worked the evening shift, which left my sister and me holding tickets to a roller coaster ride called "Nights with Dad." Every day was an adventure, seldom two in a row alike, always dependent upon his moods, and equal parts exhilarating and terrifying.

Dad giving up his day job was the first brick to crumble in the wall of denial and semblance of normal that he and my mother had attempted to create. They married in 1965, when Mom was only seventeen. She finished school by mail, since married women weren't permitted to walk the graduation ceremony. My sister was born two years later, and by 1970 they had two little girls and moved into an upstairs apartment of a house where they would live for the remainder of their life together.

Dad always knew he might get sick. He originally got cold feet about the wedding, and he told Mom they shouldn't go through with it because there was a terrible disease in his family that was going to get him and could be passed down to their future children too. But Mom wasn't hearing it. The date was set, the dress was bought, and she didn't care about something that might happen countless years in the future.

Huntington's disease was whispered about as "It" amongst Dad's mother and her four sisters: Harriet, Eilene,

Luanne, and May, before it was matched with a scientific name. Prior to increased genetic research, national awareness efforts, and community support organizations, this illness of mysterious origin was cloaked in secrecy and shame. Those affected looked drunk or crazy as the disease progressed, symptoms which left more questions than answers. If this wasn't Parkinson's, what was it? Could you catch it, or worse yet, pass it on?

My great-grandfather was born in 1893, and although he wasn't diagnosed during his lifetime, it would later be determined that he had suffered from Huntington's disease. His symptoms were mild, and they started in his 60's. Lots of old guys had a tremor, so it wasn't until two of his daughters also started showing signs, that the siblings sought answers and began to learn more about this illness that was infiltrating their family.

Great Aunt Luanne was the first sister to exhibit physical symptoms, and she did so at an early age. She declined swiftly to the point of needing long-term care. Great Aunt Eilene would develop HD later in her life and would be cared for at home by her husband until she passed away. May, Grandma, and Harriet, with no test and no cure, married and raised their families, all the while looking over their shoulders, waiting for the other shoe to drop.

Dad called HD "The Shakes" and vacillated between giving up and giving it the middle finger. Most days he was flipping HD off and living his life, with my big sister and me in the backseat along for the ride.

When my dad was in his late twenties to early thirties, he began exhibiting what we now know to be many of the physical and psychological symptoms of Huntington's disease. The early physical signs could have been interpreted as nervous twitches, habitual gestures, or simply being fidgety. At that time and even today, his psychological behaviors could be seen as depression, anger management issues, anxiety, or insomnia. Without a genetic history and limited research and education in the topic, it would have been unlikely to assume a person's conduct and emotional state were the result of a neurological condition.

When Dad dated Mom, he wore a black leather jacket, heavy boots, faded blue jeans, and rode a Harley-Davidson motorcycle. He and his gang of friends slicked their hair back into greased Pompadours and sported dark sunglasses. In pictures he resembles Arthur Fonzarelli, "Fonzie," from "Happy Days." Before they got to know him, my mother's parents initially judged him a hoodlum. Hoods were characterized for their tough, take no crap exterior, so his persona fit, regardless of the gradual onset of HD.

After he and my mom married, they both grew their hair out in the hippy fashion, and they bought an AMC Gremlin with limited edition Levi Strauss seats. I thought denim on your car seats was the coolest thing except for in the dead heat of summer, when those snaps could brand the back of your thigh if you weren't careful when getting in. After dad's hair became a shag, he got John Denver glasses, and that is the way I remember him for always, stuck in the 70's with wild hair and wire glasses, forever sliding down his nose.

Huntington's disease was originally called Huntington's Chorea, derived from the Greek word "choreia", translated "dance." Others called it Saint Vitus' dance, after the patron saint in Christian tradition who had cured a child of such an illness. But HD is so much more than a movement disorder.

In my earliest memories, Dad had tics. His arms moved constantly, as if he were stretching, warming up for a race or a tennis match. He shrugged his shoulders and cleared his throat repeatedly. He swiped his long hair back over his forehead and pushed his glasses up with the tip of his finger or by wrinkling his nose. He performed many of these actions in one synchronized movement, so that they appeared intentional. When Dad was standing, he shifted back and forth as if rocking a baby or dancing to a slow song. When walking, his gait was slightly unsteady, but he consciously, or perhaps unconsciously, compensated for that by turning it into a purposeful swagger.

Huntington's Chorea was eventually modified in name to Huntington's disease, because not all affected individuals develop chorea, and many people experience significant mood swings, strained relationships, and difficulty in mental processing well before any physical manifestation of the illness. Often called "the world's cruelest disease", according to the HDSA, Huntington's disease is described as having ALS, Parkinson's, and Alzheimer's simultaneously.

My dad's anger and erratic behavior was assumed for years to be "that's just your father." His own lack of awareness, or anosognosia, contributed to this conclusion, and his physical movements progressed so slowly, that we became accustomed to them unless taken out of our typical setting or viewed through other people's eyes. Our family, not unlike other families, learned by trial and error how to operate within our unique ecosystem.

CHAPTER 4
Lipton Soup

The key to peace in the house was keeping quiet and not causing trouble, and I learned at a young age to tiptoe and take care of myself. I was supposed to be napping, but hunger took over my fear of getting caught, and I snuck out of bed for a snack.

I watched steam rise from the trickle of water flowing from our bathroom faucet. The sink was not too high, and I could reach the handles if I climbed onto the radiator next to it and leaned over. The bathroom water got the hottest if you waited patiently. I had been warned many times by my parents that it could burn me, but I knew how to be careful.

Slowly and quietly, I ripped the packet of dry soup mix and poured the contents from the envelope into my favorite mug, which had a heart and the comic strip character Ziggy on the front, waving with his sad but winsome smile.

I held the mug under the stream, watching it fill and the

powder begin to dissolve. When it reached the top, I pulled the mug out from under the spout, not too full, lest I spill, and all heck would break loose.

With two hands I set it carefully on the board which covered the radiator and functioned as a bench. Then I turned the faucet off and focused my attention on the almost soup. I took my spoon and gently stirred, not too fast, no spilling. I broke up the remaining dry bubbles which floated on the surface, and the soup took on a yellowish, congealed consistency.

Presto, cream of chicken soup. There wasn't really any chicken to be found, but it tasted like it and the warmth was satisfying. The only thing to complain about was the little pieces of dried parsley that floated at the top, because they stuck in my teeth. If I didn't stir thoroughly, the dry bubbles would turn into mushy globs at the bottom, but that was my own fault.

This was a lunch I could do myself, nobody needed bothering. No poking the bear.

CHAPTER 5
Fisher-Price Hideaway

Despite my culinary skills in the bathroom, I had a shortcoming in what you would expect of the bathroom, the staying dry downstairs department. With Mom working the late shift and Dad seldom home in the afternoons, it was my job to nap quietly while she rested before work. If I slipped out of my room to try for a snack and woke Mom, there would be hell to pay. She'd caught me more than once monkeying around, and you didn't want that. I'd lay there waiting for my big sister to walk home from school while the clock hands crawled. The afternoons were long and boring, and if I did manage to fall asleep, I would inevitably wet the bed.

"Ugh, gross!" my sister grumbled when she came home and found me sitting on our bedroom rug in a T-shirt, wrapped in my blanket.

"Why do you have to wet the bed all the time? You think

I want to come home from school every day and change you?"

She dropped her book bag on the floor and yanked the fitted sheet and blanket off the double bed that we shared, then balled it up and hid the whole mess amongst a load of dirty towels in the laundry room, which was off our bedroom.

I didn't apologize. I didn't say anything, simply looked up at her, and her eyes softened.

"All right, all right, let's find something for you to wear."

She dug in our dresser drawer and yanked out some underwear and hand-me-down blue jeans. I pulled them on quickly.

"Where are your wet underpants? You better not have anything else hidden around here, or Mom's going to kill you!" she threatened.

She began scouting around under the bed and behind the toys, and her eyes lit on the Fisher-Price Barn.

"No! Don't look in there, there's nothing in there." I pleaded, which was of course a dead giveaway that there was indeed something in there.

The Fisher-Price Play Family Barn was my favorite toy, complete with a tractor, barn doors that made a "moo" sound when opened, and a collection of plastic farm animals, including a horse, cow, pigs, and sheep. The barn doors closed with a swinging latch, the rooster and chicken were stored in the upper coop, and it had a handle on top from which I carried it everywhere I went. My sister knew from experience that I stashed all matter of collectibles in my barn.

She pulled impatiently at the hinge.

"Moo," went the barn door.

She made a face. "Lori!"

I shrunk smaller as she extracted a bologna sandwich wrapped in toilet paper. The white bread was tough, and the meat smelled bad, evidence that the lunch had been hidden in the barn for several days.

Next, she made for the chicken coop, sliding the plastic doors open. Her eyes were murderous as she took the toilet paper from the sandwich and used it to extract my wet underpants from their hiding spot. Pinching them between two fingers, she carried them like roadkill to the laundry room and buried them deeper in the pile.

"What is wrong with you?" she asked.

I couldn't answer, but I knew to wait it out until her anger cooled, and then we might go outside to play. She always forgave me.

When a young child stows away food, they may be stressed or food insecure, worried about their next meal. When a child conceals bedwetting or bathroom accidents, they may be ashamed or coping with anxiety. I'm not sure what psychologists would say about a little girl combining both in one storage location, but I was nothing if not resourceful.

CHAPTER 6
Kid Duty

Throughout my school years Dad still drove the car. I had no other frame of reference, and therefore knew nothing different or out of the ordinary about his driving skills. His foot shifted on the pedal, alternating between slow and then fast, and his speed seemed to vary based on his mood. He adjusted the dials on the radio, cranked his window up and down, and was in constant movement in the driver seat, but this never deterred his daily outings.

Sometimes he left early in the morning, other days he slept until noon if he had been up late the previous night, but he always went somewhere. Dad had typical routes which involved the back roads of rural Southern Wisconsin, and until my sister was deemed old enough to stay home alone and watch me, we came along on most of Dad's travel that took place at night.

"Get in the van!" Dad called from the driveway one night.

He stood with the driver's side door open in his standard attire of cutoff jeans and T-shirt, jingling his keys. My sister and I were playing in the backyard.

We scrambled off the "boat," which was a large crumbling cement porch that jutted out from the downstairs unit and served as our ship, bringing countless hours of imaginative fun. Avoiding the sharks in the water, we hopped down and made haste. Dad didn't like stragglers, and an evening ride held the promise of adventure.

Dad was on kid duty weeknights while Mom worked the PM shift, and during the warmer months of the year, we'd often take a drive before bedtime. The destination was never revealed ahead of time, and we would ride quietly in anticipation.

Occasionally he would make slow laps around the town square which circled the courthouse. When this happened my sister and I held our breath, praying he didn't pull into a parking spot to talk to his old neighborhood friend Trucker. Trucker worked in a lower-level shop, and Dad had to descend a flight of basement stairs to see him. Those two could easily go back and forth for an hour or more while we waited in the car, windows rolled down a crack.

Another regular downtown stop was to an upper room bar called Dirty John's which was smoky and dark but better than waiting for Dad and Trucker to wrap it up. My sister and I would spin on stools and get called dolls by the bartender. We would drink Shirley Temples while we belted out the chorus to country songs like "Lucille" and "Mammas Don't Let Your Babies Grow Up to Be Cowboys."

Things looked up if we headed towards either of the baseball diamonds in town. My dad would watch a softball game or two while we made a run for the playground equipment and, on a good night, were each given a nickel to spend at the candy stand.

At the games Dad always perched at the top-most bleacher, clutching a waxed paper cup of RC Cola, and I constantly worried about him falling or spilling his drink on the spectators seated below. I detected something wasn't right because my dad didn't look or act like other dads. He shifted and staggered, his arms swung around of their own accord, and he cleared his throat and snorted loudly. The bleachers themselves would shift and shimmy under his movements, and sometimes people stared, which made my face feel hot.

CHAPTER 7
Cadiz Springs

The best outcome of evening drives was when Dad's travel route took us out of town towards the country backroads. He would stop at the liquor mart to pick up some "brewskies" for later, weave his way through town and then keep going. This path meant Cadiz Springs or what Dad called Zander's Lake and a whole evening of delicious freedom.

Cadiz Springs State Recreation Area is a state park unit of Wisconsin, featuring two reservoirs on a spring-fed creek, which Dad claimed was his "church" whenever he got grief from Mom for not attending. The park is known for its two lakes, Beckman and Zander, which are man-made reservoirs created by damming up Zander Creek. If I could summarize the happiest of any day in my years growing up it would be a day spent at Cadiz.

Dad would pull into the parking lot and remind us to stick close. Then he'd make for the hiking trail which ran the perimeter of the lake, while we played on the toys and explored the forest.

On some occasions we were invited to come along on the trek around the lake. There were rules, though. You had to find a good hiking stick, you had to keep up, and you had to be quiet. It was also a package deal. We had to come together because he wouldn't let the other one stay behind alone. At times, my sister and I would argue about whether we would go or not, but we usually agreed it was worth it, or she trumped the decision with older sister status.

We grabbed our sticks and hurried up, because even with his meandering cadence, he still took three steps to each of our ones. If we were especially good, Dad would get a sly smile and suggest that there might be pennies hidden along the trail by the Leprechauns. I don't know how that man did it. I thought myself a perceptive child, continuously on the lookout for trouble brewing and how to deescalate it, and yet he was either planting those pennies ahead of time on his daily circumference of the lake, or he was stealth enough to get out ahead of us and hide them on the fly. The coins were not in plain sight either, you had to hunt, step off the groomed path and peek behind oak trees. I'd find decaying trunks with mossy lichen growing, and there, sure enough, would be a shiny coin. I'd spy one, scoop it up, and stick it in my pocket. When I looked over at Dad, he'd be smiling.

Further around the path, we would come to what Dad

called the "Tabletop," which were limestone outcroppings of flat rocks, and if it was a warm day we'd lie there like a pride of lions and soak in the sun.

Dad taught us which plants were safe to eat. He let us pick the Red Clover, pull their little purple tubes out of the blossom, and suck the sweetness. He foraged for Morel mushrooms while we picked giant puffballs and gooseberries.

He showed us every bird and duck, identifying them all by name, and let us spot the turtles sunning themselves on fallen logs sticking up out of the water. The highlight of the day for him would be if a hawk circled overhead. He'd point it out, and we would stand still looking up and gazing at it until it banked, and with a shrill cry headed out of sight. My dad would watch that Red-tailed hawk until it disappeared, his eyes wistful as if he wanted to grow wings and fly away with it. Eventually he would gather himself and say, "let's go," and we would follow him back.

On the nights that we chose to stay and play on the playground equipment we had free reign except for the waterfront and beach area. When we got thirsty, my sister and I combined both our strengths, raising the pump handle up and down to draw metallic water from the spigot. We spent hours in the woods, collecting acorns and making stick families complete with stick babies wrapped up in fuzzy Lamb's-ears, their soft leaves making the perfect fleece blankets. As the sun began to set, we would find our way back to the van.

Dad was forever talking the ear off the lifeguard at the beach, and we usually had to wait for him to finish, his arms waving dramatically. He held onto the leg of her raised wooden chair for balance, and she would gaze down at him when she wasn't watching the swimmers. I was embarrassed, but not sure why. She smiled and listened politely, but I could tell that her smile wasn't genuine.

He would wind down like a watch and eventually meet us at the van. The ride home would go one of two ways. If Dad was in a good mood, he would take a right out of the parking lot, and I knew we were headed to Franklin Road, with the best bumps and hills. We would initially ramble along, and then he'd speed up and take the dips like an amusement park ride while we squealed as our stomachs dropped.

If Dad still wasn't done, we'd find Smock Valley Road and shoot down the slopes and turns like Olympic skiers. The whole time we were careening the curves we'd have to be ready for a sudden stop, as Dad would pull over on a moment's notice to point out and count the deer he spotted in the farm fields and wood lines.

Only when we sensed the good mood prevailed would my sister and I beg him for "Rudy the Elephant" stories. He would think for a minute, one hand on the wheel, gazing out the window, and then begin. He told crazy tales about a little elephant named Rudy who went on all sorts of journeys and explorations, got himself in a fix a time or two, but always resolved at the end. I once said he should write the stories down in a book, but he reminded us that he didn't read and couldn't write.

If Dad's temperament had shifted, the ride was quiet, and somehow my sister and I knew the difference, me more than her, but both of us had radar for whether it was okay to ask for a Rudy story or best to sit still in the back seat and not cause any trouble.

On those nights, we would sometimes drive fast, but then it was an angry fast followed by a sad slow. If my stomach tickled with a hill, I knew not to shout out or beg him to go faster, and if I had to go to the bathroom and he was putting along, I knew to hold it without complaining.

We would eventually find our way home, usually by the fastest route, and then it was off to bed without any arguing. I don't remember there ever being a difference on whether it was a school night or not. It was all about Dad's mood.

CHAPTER 8
Madtown

It was the weekend, and Mom and Dad were getting along. I could tell because there was no fighting, no door slamming, and no awful, tense silent treatment. They were cuddling and talking softly, which was so rare that it noticeably changed the atmosphere of the apartment. On a weekend when Mom didn't have to work and these kinds of stars aligned, Dad would talk her into coming along on a trip, and the whole family would go for a longer distance than our regular nightly outings.

This could be good or bad, depending on whether the feel-good mood lasted for the entire journey. Extended trips made me especially nervous, because it was a longer time for everyone to manage; however, these outings could be fun because they often involved going to Madison, which Dad called "Madtown."

Madison was our closest big city, with tall buildings, highways, and shopping malls. Hitting a scale of ten out of ten was a trip to the Madison Zoo, and on a best day ever, he stopped at Vilas Beach before heading home.

Today was a Madison day. I heard them talking about it over breakfast, and when we got in the car and headed out on Highway 69, I knew it was going to happen. I sat quietly in the back and tried not to fidget or touch my sister to prevent her from yelling at me and ruining anything. Dad fiddled with the radio and rolled the window up and down throughout the trip, but Mom didn't get irritated, no huffy breathes at all. Sometimes I pulled out a joke or tried to steer the conversation, but none of this damage control was necessary today.

We cruised past the Belleville turn off, made our way through Paoli, and entered Madison via the Beltline on the west side. I tensed, as a few miles of the Highway 12 Beltline with idiots who were born yesterday might tank our trip, but Dad gunned the gas, merged into traffic, and kept a steady pace until our exit.

Just before the zoo Dad hung a left at Lake Wingra to check out the Arboretum. The trees hung over the road like a canopy, and sunlight dappled through the branches. Dad rolled his window down again, this time all the way, and the breeze blew my hair around. I could smell the sweet scent of decaying leaves.

My dad drove slow in the Arboretum, but it was okay because everyone is supposed to drive slow there, and no one got mad if you swerved around a bit or stopped to look at something of interest. I only worried about him veering too close to the bikers or joggers, who were everywhere.

The University of Wisconsin Madison Arboretum is considered the birthplace of ecological restoration and is thriving yet today. With a 1200-acre teaching and research facility, the Arboretum conserves and restores land, advances science, and offers both public outreach and community involvement. All I knew at my age was that this 2-mile loop was a tonic for Dad, and I witnessed it visibly calming and restoring him.

He turned around at the ending cul-de-sac, and we made our way back through, crawling along as slowly as the first leg. As we approached the stop sign at the exit, I held my breath. He paused, and when I just about thought that he was going to make a right turn and head back home, he turned left and coasted into the zoo parking lot. He cut the engine, and we climbed out of the car and headed to the gate.

The Henry Vilas Zoo in Dane County has been around for over a hundred years. It is one of the only remaining free admission public zoos in America, and my dad was an expert on every animal that lived there. As we navigated the zoo, there was a certain path we always took and a specific amount of time we spent at each exhibit, no deviations allowed. Dad liked to see the seals, then walk over to the giraffes and camels, and then head through to the African lions' pen, where he'd huff at the male until the king "oofed" back.

Dad saved what he deemed the best for last, the bears, big brown bears and mammoth polars. The joint bear enclosures were made of stone, with iron fencing surrounding them and a trench many feet deep separating us from them. At the very bottom of that cavernous pit were ball caps, toddler toys, and frisbees, things people had dropped accidentally, or litter tossed on purpose, never to be retrieved.

Other people were looking at the bears too, waving their arms, trying to get them to talk or stand up and do tricks, because these bears did do tricks. They had an assortment of half deflated basketballs and volleyballs, and they would stand up on their hind legs and bat them back and forth with each other, much to the delight of the onlookers.

Dad slipped a sly smile at us and pulled a bag of jumbo marshmallows from his side pocket. There was a sign posted on the fence that read "Do NOT Feed the Bears!" but this sign didn't apply to my dad. Dad shook the marshmallow bag, and it made a crinkle and a rustle, causing the people around us to notice. Some seemed interested in what Dad was up to, but others gave an indignant look that said "Can't you read? You're not following the rules!"

Dad gave them a look back that said, "Mind your own beeswax!"

He pulled out a marshmallow, held it high in the air and hollered at the Papa Grizzly.

"Get up. Sit up, now!"

I swear that bear knew my dad's voice. He turned slowly, looked us over, and plopped down on his big hairy behind, raising his front paws in the air. Dad chucked the marshmallow over his head in a high arc, and the bear caught it mid-air, gobbling it down.

Now this group gathered wasn't so forehead wrinkled.

Now there was an audience ready for a show, and Dad was happy to oblige. Marshmallow after marshmallow soft balled into the air, and he had those bears pawing and juggling their toys, balancing like they were performing in the circus.

My stomach hurt. I worried that the Zookeeper would appear and yell at us. I also worried that the crowd would judge us or tattle, but at the same time I felt proud that my dad could train bears at the zoo. The stirring swirl of worry soup in my stomach got the best of the proud feeling in my chest, and I pulled on Mom's sleeve.

"I have to go to the bathroom," I said to her.

She frowned and huffed, as if I was ruining everything, and told my father that she had to take me.

"Show's over," Dad said and tucked the rest of the marshmallows back in his jacket.

"Sorry, Dad," I said, but he affectionately scrubbed the top of my head.

"It's all right, kiddo. They've had enough."

After I'd gone to the bathroom, we made our way to the exit gates, as it was time to head home. We pulled out of the lot, and even though we didn't stop at the beach that day, this had been a successful trip, and for that I was grateful.

I dozed off in the back seat on the way home and woke up groggy as we entered the city limits. If I faked sleep until the driveway, I was still young enough to be carried upstairs to my room, so I closed my eyes tightly and kept even breaths.

"Mom, she's not really asleep! She's pretending!" my sister yelled, trying to out me as the overhead dome lights came on and everyone gathered their things.

"It's okay, I got her," Dad said.

Dad scooped me up and settled me against his shoulder as he climbed the green steps. On a scale of ten this scored an eleven, better than the beach.

CHAPTER 9
House Rules

I dried the dishes, wiping them as quickly and quietly as I could, making sure to get each plate dry. The only light on was above the kitchen sink. The tv blared in the other room, and Dad was sprawled on the couch, a bowl of chips balancing on the arm. I moved on to the silverware, then glassware.

I was almost done when, Crash!

Oh no, why did that have to happen? And tonight, of all nights, when things weren't going especially well already.

Fear crept around my insides and knotted its way into my middle. I thought I might be sick, but I was too paralyzed to make for the bathroom.

I waited for the response I knew was coming. I didn't think he would hit me, but I was never sure. Adrenaline coursed through my body, and I cringed at his inevitable wrath.

"Don't move!" he bellowed from the living room, hauled himself up from the chair, and stomped into the kitchen.

He ordered me to sit on the floor in one spot and keep still. I sat cross-legged, holding the damp dishtowel. He made me put on a pair of his socks so I wouldn't cut my bare feet, and they slumped on my legs.

The lecture went on for what felt like hours, his voice rising and falling with emotion, angry and full of loudness, then quiet and full of sadness. Tears came. He cried because I didn't care enough to do my job the right way, then kept crying and said Mom didn't love us and no wonder. He screamed at me again and told me it was my fault because I was careless.

Dad brought out every cleaning supply we owned and began sweeping the floor, gathering the shattered glass into a dustpan, and brushing it into the garbage can. He turned on every light in the whole house, and it was strange to see the rooms so abnormally bright. He vacuumed for what seemed like an hour, around and around my statue body.

His voice ebbed and flowed over the sound of the vacuum. I felt myself falling asleep, as it was very late, but he woke me, yelling and cursing that the least I could do was stay awake, since he was doing all the work.

What had I done to bring on this anger? I had broken one of the drinking glasses, but more importantly I had broken one of the rules, and there were so many: don't make loud noises, don't spill your drink, don't talk on the phone. We couldn't prepare meals in the kitchen, and we weren't allowed to change the tv channel or open any windows. My older sister couldn't use hairspray or perfume, we couldn't shut the door when we took a bath, no one was ever invited into the house, and no one could answer the door if anyone stopped by.

The rules went on and on, and they changed like the wind. All the little rules added up to a singular big one, the last thing Mom commanded each night before she went to work: "Don't upset your father!" Our family operated under this mission statement, and it was top-secret and classified, because all our members were to carry it out as if everything was fine.

The yelling gave way to silence, and this was almost the worst part. Could I get up and go? Dare I try? My legs were numb. He looked at me, with such an expression of hurt and disappointment and said, "Go on, get out of here."

I grabbed my opportunity to escape and scurried off on pins and needles legs, hoping I was asleep before Mom arrived, before the yelling started again.

CHAPTER 10
Diving

I curled my toes vice-like into his tan, wet shoulders. My knees were shaking.

"Hold my thumbs," he instructed, and I did, as if I was about to ride in the rodeo.

"Now, stand up," he said.

I stood, high above the water, the breeze sending shivers through the late afternoon sun. I clutched a meaty thumb on each side, my hands barely forming fists around them.

"Now, when I count to three, I want you to let go and dive forward." He made this sound as natural as tying your shoe, not like he was going to send his little girl plunging headfirst into our backyard pool.

"Here we go! One. two. three. DIVE!"

He sprung out of the water and ducked his head forward to boost me air born. I knew if I didn't let go of his thumbs I would probably wind up with dislocated shoulders and a nose full of water, so I released my grip and plunged forward into the deep. It was sort of a dive-belly-flop hybrid, and I felt the sting as I heard the splash.

When I surfaced, Dad smiled and said, "Okay, let's try it again."

We'd been at this for a while now, not long after he decided that I needed to know how to dive. I'd been swimming since I was four, and I was a little fish according to my dad, who would know. Growing up in our town, he became famous for spending afternoons at the city pool, performing back flips, double somersaults, and all sorts of stunts off the boards. According to Dad's stories, he was a legend, and crowds gathered to watch on the day he attempted a two-and-a-half gainer.

Since my older sister still plugged her nose when going under, Dad decided that I would be the one to advance my swimming abilities. In most of life, he bypassed her and granted the athletic and boyish events to me, his second girl who was supposed to be his son. I played the role, drinking in the sporadic affection it brought. I would have grown a moustache had it garnered me praise from this man, so, despite my apprehension, I clamored back up on his shoulders for another go at the skill of diving. He paused and looked up at me with a sneaky twinkle in his eye.

"You know, I bet if you could learn how to dive by the

end of the day, your piggy bank might be full of bubble gum tomorrow."

I couldn't believe my ears. Bubble gum! It sounded way too good to be true. Like the kitten he brought home last spring as our new pet, only to mysteriously disappear two days later, never to be mentioned again. Like the vacation we started out on earlier this summer, only to have Dad get mad at the born yesterday driver ahead of us for cutting him off. He turned around, bringing us right back home. Disappointment was a constant companion in my house, and the only way to avoid it was to anticipate it and adjust my expectations accordingly.

But a small flame of trust, a pilot light of hope deep down inside of me flickered with his words, and this time I dove off his shoulders in almost perfect form. My hands prayed above my head, and I met the water with little to no mark. He was applauding and grinning when I bobbed up for air.

"That's my girl," he said, "We're done for today."

We climbed out of the pool and went inside. The rest of the evening passed without excitement. My sister was quiet because Dad was bragging on me about the diving. I downplayed it because I didn't want her to feel bad, and because when she was mad at me, she ignored me, and that was the worst.

Dad was in a good mood the rest of the night, going around the house singing silly songs. He even made dinner and let us drink RC Cola with our SpaghettiOs.

When he sent us to bed Dad said, "Don't forget to check your bank tomorrow 'Little Fish'."

Embarrassed, I smiled and climbed into bed. I wished he wouldn't talk about it anymore. I didn't dare get excited because it hurt too badly when dreams got broken.

My coin bank was a fuzzy grey rabbit with glass eyes just like my sister's. We both had gotten them for Christmas, and it felt like those rabbit eyes were staring at me while I tried to settle in. I couldn't sleep, so I practiced in my head how I would act and what I would say in the morning when the gum was not there. I drifted off deciding that the best thing to do would be to pretend that I had forgotten too. It was no big deal.

But in the morning, there it was. I rubbed sleep out of my eyes and sat up, throwing off the covers. My bank was crammed full of Bazooka Joe, and what didn't fit in the rabbit was spilling out onto the top of the dresser. It was the pink penny gum, the kind in the waxy paper with all the powder leaking out, that was so soft and so sweet it made your teeth hurt if you held it between your molars for too long. The kind with the cartoon on the inside, cartoons that never were very funny, but you always unfolded the wrapper and read them anyway.

I stood in my pajamas and stared at that gum, and when Dad came in, he just laughed and laughed. He must have thought my surprised look was so funny, but all his amusement made me even more nervous. Dad had a bit of a mean streak. I was afraid he might be laughing because the gum wasn't real, or he was going to take it away or something. Signals fired and misfired in my brain.

"Go on, have a piece!" he urged, although we hadn't even had breakfast yet.

I took one, and it was delicious, just as sugary, and yummy as gum should be. I offered one to my sister.

"No thanks," she said in front of Dad, but then accepted one after he left the room, still chuckling to himself.

I sat there on my bed chewing and thinking. This bank full of gum had messed with my entire system of how things worked around here. This was the first promise I remember Dad had ever kept. If he started keeping all his promises, would our lives change completely? Would he get a job? Would he sleep at night and not get so angry anymore? How was I ever to stop myself from hoping again?

CHAPTER 11
Homemade Inventions and Store-Bought Defeat

The pool I earned my gum in was just one of many swimming pools Dad built in our backyard over the years. Although RC Colas and SpaghettiOs were considered luxuries, in the dog days of southern Wisconsin's high heat and humidity, my father deemed pools a necessity. Every summer that man was dreaming up new ways to create swimming holes, with most of his inventions being homemade improvisations, involving plastic sheeting, cement bricks, and a lot of swearing when they busted loose, releasing tidal waves onto the crispy grass.

One of his better projects initially looked like a winner, after he had been drawing up plans for days. He built it into what we called "the ditch," a steep downward sloping side of our yard that bordered the concrete wall of the cement factory next door. It was a deep, ready-made hole, and all he had to do was line it with plastic, brace it and fill it with the hose. Soon "the ditch" was rippling with cool clear water, and my sister and I were paddling around like tadpoles.

Dad kicked back in his lawn chair in the driveway, visibly pleased. I was proud of him too, and I wished there was a spot to mark this day as a good one, a day of accomplishment.

Unfortunately, this trench had historically been a place where garbage was dumped and then buried. We later discovered that if you dug down a couple of feet you hit all sorts of foreign objects better left covered up.

That afternoon, as I swam down to the bottom, my kneecap connected with a broken bottle, the sharp glass poking through the plastic of the floor lining. I surfaced with blood running down my leg and a gash that set my head spinning when I found the source. My sister started screaming.

I've never seen Dad look so serious. He acted like a dad on TV as he calmly wrapped my leg in a towel, positioned me, still dripping, in the car and sped to the hospital, shirtless and in his cut-off blue jeans.

Dad was talking a mile a minute to the lady at the counter, and by the time we checked in, I was shivering in my wet bathing suit and towel. The nurse lifted me onto a big steel table, and we waited for the doctor. She asked me a lot of questions, and I told her all about our homemade pools and how I cut my knee, trying to explain more clearly because Dad hadn't been making any sense at all. Her lips pressed into a straight little line while she listened to my description of "the ditch" and how it was a perfect location minus the broken beer bottle.

"My dad said, 'It's like it was asking to be a swimming pool!'," I said proudly.

She made some notes on a clipboard, patted me on the back, and gave me a bright smile. The doctor came in all business, and the nurse wiped yellow goop on my knee with a cotton ball.

"Now this is going to sting a little," she admitted, "but I want you to hold my hand and squeeze it real tight, can you do that?"

I nodded my head vigorously, as I wished to please this woman, and I also needed to be tough for my dad. I didn't want to cry and ruin all the happiness of his latest pool invention. I hoped that if I could be tough through this, we could head back home and still take another swim before bed time.

As the stitches went in, I watched with wide eyes. It was like someone else's knee there on the table, the needle piercing my skin like cloth as the doctor sewed me up. The nurse sucked in her breath as I wrung the blood from her hand. Eight stitches later, we were done.

"Wow, you were a real trooper!" the nurse said, rubbing life back into her hand. "And you even watched!"

I shrugged and grinned as if to say, "Yeah, I do this all the time."

Dad looked on, subdued, his animation depleted, and the

earlier excitement of pool triumph had drained from his face. He scribbled his signature on the forms, not saying another word until we exited through the automatically sliding doors.

"You were brave in there, kid." He messed up my damp hair as he carried me to the car.

Back home, Dad took the ditch pool apart, even as I protested and promised that I would be more careful and not go down as deep. He was defeated, and all the bravery in the world wasn't going to change that.

I thought back yard pools would never happen for us again, but later that summer Dad came home with a big cardboard box and renewed energy. This store-bought pool was a put-together kit, with a real pump, a vinyl cover, and a ladder to climb in and out. It was the best one yet, but we had it up only that one summer and then, as suddenly as Dad's pool building obsession had begun, it ended. He said he just didn't feel like putting them up anymore, and we were done swimming in the backyard.

CHAPTER 12
Secret Clinic Visit with Grandma

My sister and I rode in the back seat of Grandma's big pink Cadillac. Grandma wore a genuine fur overcoat and carried a large leather purse. Her jet-black hair was teased up in a beehive, and her red lipstick matched the polish on her long fingernails. My grandma was heavy set, but she was flowy and glamorous, reminding me of a movie star from the 1950's. Riding in the Cadillac was like rolling on waves as we floated through town.

"Where are we going, Grandma?" I asked her.

"Oh, we're just going for a little clinic visit," she replied nonchalantly, with that forever smile on her face. "We're going to have a test, and the test will help the scientists fix the disease in our family."

I felt like I had swallowed an ice cube, as a cold and dark sensation formed in the middle of my stomach. I knew she was talking about Huntington's disease. It would come up occasionally, and sometimes Grandpa would shush her. Other times, he'd let her talk. Grandma was convinced that she had Huntington's disease like her father, who I had never met. She had been doing research and was now a member of an association. I didn't know what an association was, but she said it was going to get some answers.

My dad called Grandma a "crazy old bat," and while he loved her dearly, he wasn't going to listen to any of that hocus pocus about the "Heebie Jeebies."

When we arrived at the clinic, Grandma slowly climbed out of the driver's seat and led us through the entrance and up to the registration desk. She spoke to the woman behind the counter for a few minutes, who first looked serious and then smiled at my sister and me. She pointed in the direction of the elevators.

We entered the elevators and rode to the third floor, where we spoke to another woman behind another counter who looked serious and then smiled at us again. This time the woman behind the counter passed papers to Grandma that she clutched in her hands, and we sat together in the waiting room.

Grandma told me and my sister that we could look at the children's books that were on the table, but I said I was okay. Eventually our names were called, and we obediently followed a lady in a white coat. Grandma handed her the papers, and the lady in the white coat pinned them to her clipboard.

She then introduced herself as the lab technician and sat me down in a chair with an arm rest. "This is only going to be a little pinch," she said, while gathering a needle and some plastic tubes. I was terrified. I had no idea that I was going to have to have blood drawn.

She gave a reassuring smile, and I didn't want to argue or go against Grandma, so I sat quietly. It did so much more than pinch. She shoved the needle in my arm, pulled out my blood, and collected it in three test tubes, one after the other. Then she dropped those tubes in an envelope and sealed it shut.

She undid the heavy rubber band that was cutting off my circulation and put a Sylvester and Tweety Band-Aid over the spot where she had sucked the blood. Then she gave me a sucker, and it was over. My sister came out of a similar room with a Mickey Mouse Band-Aid on her arm, also sucking on a sucker. We looked at each other as if we had just shared the same experience, but had no idea why, except for an inkling that we had participated in some research. We shared the same conclusion as well: Dad was gonna be pissed.

Grandma guided us back to the elevator, and perhaps she read our minds.

"Girls, we're not going to talk to your father about this, okay?" she held both of our gazes.

We both nodded, our sucker sticks moving up and down with our heads.

"Now, who wants ice cream from the Dairy Queen?" Grandma asked.

Yes. Our heads nodded in synchronicity once again. Dairy Queen sounded really good.

CHAPTER 13
Sleeping on "The Green"

"**I** hate you!" my sister yelled at him.

"I'm not real crazy about you either, 'Bony Moronie'," he replied in a calmer but scarier voice. "But if you slam that bedroom door again, it'll be the last time it hangs on its hinges. I'll rip the damn thing off."

"Don't call me that! And I need privacy!" she shot back.

They were at it again. My sister and Dad circled the ring in multiple rounds on any given night. The topic would be any actions causing strong and bad smells according to Dad, such as spraying perfume, using hair spray, or painting your nails, all ordinary activities that tweens were obsessed with. Additional fuel for the fire was the iron rule that our shared bedroom door must remain open for air flow, even if we were changing, so we dressed hastily or ducked into the closet for discretion. We also weren't allowed to talk on the phone with friends and absolutely could not have anyone over to our house.

My dad, who claimed he couldn't read but likely possessed a fourth or fifth-grade level, had somehow mastered alliteration and christened his girls "Bony Moronie" and "Booper Magoo." His creativity was lost on us, as we hated the nicknames, but the more we fussed, the more he enjoyed it.

When we were little, Dad would twirl my sister and channel Larry Williams, shuffling around the living room singing that he had a girl called "Bony Moronie," who was as skinny as a stick of macaroni. As my sister entered her teen years, she remained slender and would stay that way most of her life, but she did not find this nickname a compliment, even when it was used in affection.

As the story is told, when I was a preschooler Dad would sit my tiny behind on the palm of his hand and circle me around the house to carousel music. "Boop, boop, boop, boop." Dad would sing, and I would giggle and ask him to go faster and higher. Even though "Booper Magoo" got its legs from boop-boop rides and sweet dad-daughter time, I was also dreadfully embarrassed by this nickname, but I somehow sensed that reacting to it only egged him on and limited my comments.

I overheard enough of tonight's context to learn that my sister had tried to cook something for dinner and must not have done it right, violating yet another rule. Dad wouldn't tolerate making meals that resulted in any kind of mess, the kitchen being basically off-limits. Anything we did in there got in his way, smelled bad, was too loud, or caused a change that got under his skin. Most evenings if we couldn't heat something quickly before he got home from his regular outing, we had to wait until later at night and make a cold sandwich when he was soaking in the bathtub.

How did I know the secret to avoiding the tripping of kitchen traps and all other emotional triggers? I'm not sure, but I seemed to have an internal sensor to assess the situation and determine what I could and couldn't get away with. I then acted accordingly within those boundaries.

My sister possessed no such radar and would push his buttons routinely. It almost seemed like she intentionally jumped with both feet into a big pile of conflict on any given day. They would argue, their voices getting louder, and tempers escalated. Soon things began to be thrown around and doors slammed. As she grew older, curse words added to the mix, and she sounded like Mom.

Conflict made my stomach hurt unless I could float away. Floating away, I learned later in my life, was disassociation or depersonalization, but when I was young, floating away meant to soften your eyes and look anywhere but in front of you. By focusing on one little thing in the distance, your head would get light, and your body would get floaty, and off you would go, to a place where the voices somehow were muffled, and nothing could hurt you. I would live in this place for as long as it took for the dust to settle, and then I would come back down.

The best place to float was on "The Green," which was our indoor porch, and Dad nick-named it so because of the color of the carpet. We lived on the second floor of an old house. You walked up 15 wooden outdoor steps, also painted green, to get to our inside porch, and then there were five more steps until you got to the green carpet.

"The Green" was where I spent many hours as a young girl with all my toys, playing make believe with Fisher-Price people, toy cars and tractors, and Honey Hill Bunch dolls. A part of me felt too old to be out here now, but "The Green" was where I would still curl up with my blanket and float if anyone was fighting, if Dad was pacing, or if I was waiting for Mom to get done working, like tonight.

My dad and sister must have gone to their separate corners, because it grew quiet, and as I fell asleep out there, no one even noticed that I was gone. Usually, Mom came home from working her second shift at 11:00 PM, but tonight she didn't return until 2:00 AM, because she was putting in overtime in preparation for the holiday season. Christmas time was when Mom worked lots of hours and made good money.

I heard her climbing up the steps, and I rubbed the sleep out of my eyes and sat up. She practically stumbled over me, curled up on "The Green" with my blanket and stuffed dog, Henry. Mom always smelled like Wrigley 's chewing gum and cigarette smoke, not because she smoked, but because all the other ladies on her key punch shift did, and it would rub off on her.

"What on earth are you doing out here at this hour?" She asked, in an exasperated voice.

She sounded exhausted and annoyed that I wasn't tucked in my bed, and that Dad was slacking on his job. I didn't want him to get blamed or start yet another fight, so I was quick to answer.

"I was waiting to say goodnight to you," I said.

Her voice softened, and she gave me a cuddle and a pat on the head.

"You need to get to bed, you have school tomorrow."

I waited to see if she would ask.

"Are you hungry, do you want a snack?"

My stomach growled at the idea. "Yes please."

She poured me some cereal and then shooed me off to bed. Mom always looked tired and irritated, whether from her night at work or that she had to come back to us, I was never sure which.

CHAPTER 14
Dark Magic

Sometimes Bea came at night to play with us while Mom was working, and Dad went out. Bea was Dad's cousin, and her real name was Beatrice, but he nicknamed her "Bea."

I loved her, she had a big smile, made SpaghettiOs's for dinner, and we danced to her LP records on the turn table before bedtime. My sister and I had to promise not to tell Bea's mother, Great Aunt May, that she bought them, because they were Rock-n-Roll. I joked that I was going to tell, and her eyes got wide, but I never really would.

Dad hired Bea to babysit when he went out on the town with his cousin, who had been his buddy growing up, because they were the same age. Mom always said that the two of them together were nothing but trouble.

If Bea couldn't babysit, then Dad's cousin came over to hang out and drink beer with Dad while my sister and I played in our room. Having him come over made Dad happy, but I could tell Mom wasn't really thrilled, and shortly after, he was no longer around, perhaps that was when he and his family moved out west to Colorado. Dad seemed restless with his cousin and friend gone.

Shortly after, Dad went on a diet, and his mind was laser fixed on it. He got skinnier and skinnier until there was almost nothing left of him. I often found him in front of the full-length mirror, doing karate moves and turning front to back, eyeing himself from every angle and sucking in his stomach. We would still take trips at night, to the ballpark or Cadiz Springs, but it took Dad hours of preparing in front of the mirror before we would leave.

His long hair was still feathered back, and he would take frequent swipes at it with his comb. Dad's eyes were wild, and the energy almost seemed to thrum off him. He cleared his throat constantly and made an odd clucking sound with his tongue. My sister, never one to hold back, questioned him about it one night.

"Dad, why do you make that noise?" she asked.

"What noise?" he said.

"You know, 'cluck-cluck', why do you do that all the time?" She persisted, and I winced, somehow reckoning that this was something we shouldn't ask about, but he just grunted and ignored her.

During this time when Dad was running at a heightened

frequency, I remember one night Dad called us from our room to say he had a surprise for us. When my sister and I came out, he told us that he was going to do a magic trick. He was going to float in the air, so we had to go back in our room and wait for him to call us again once he was ready.

This was both unsettling and exciting, so we returned to our room and cleaned up our toys while we waited. It wasn't long until he called us back out. I stood behind my sister, and we slowly cracked open our bedroom door. The living room was pitch black without the forever glow of the TV, and the only light came from a candle flickering on the coffee table.

Dad sat sideways on what I would learn later was a kitchen chair. He had draped a black cloth over his shoulders and body, covering the chair and puddling on the floor at his feet. He told us to watch from where we were, and then he began to hum a ghostly tune and lift his legs lengthwise while reclining his torso back, balancing on his backside.

From our angle and with the black sheet covering him, he gave every sleight of hand that he was truly floating. It was realistic enough that, when I heard my sister suck in her breath, I too believed he was hovering in the air, and I began to cry loudly.

I don't think that was the reaction he was going for, because he quickly settled himself back onto the chair and beckoned us over. My sister went, but I hung back, so he went so far as to switch on all the lights in the living room and show me how the trick worked. I dried up the tears quickly and was embarrassed to be the scaredy-cat. After all, it was just floating, and I was the expert in that, wasn't I?

As quickly and feverishly as Dad had obsessed with his diet, he dropped it. His weight would then fluctuate up and down, but mostly up for many years after. Dad remained heavy set until the involuntary movements of HD produced the "be careful what you wish for" caloric reduction for which it is known.

He returned to sleeping most days and roaming the house at night, and the intense look in his eyes faded. As mysteriously as it arrived, the clucking sound he frequently made also exited, and there were no more magic tricks.

CHAPTER 15
Acceptable Answers

Every Sunday morning, without fail, my mother packed my sister and me into the back seat of our Gremlin and drove us to the Presbyterian Church on the other side of town. My dad was a Christmas Eve church attender at best and made sniping comments the whole time we got ready, laughing, and poking fun.

My father had grown up Catholic and told us stories about attending the local parochial elementary school when he was a boy. He recounted the horrors of the nuns and their wooden rulers that they would smack down on your hands if you were fidgeting or not paying attention to the lesson. I imagined if he wiggled even half as much then as he did now, he'd be getting whacked for sure.

Dad would recite a little Latin when he wanted to show off, but he was having none of that pew sitting nonsense. Today he was in rare form.

"Dominus vobiscum! Say hi to Mother Mary and the Pope for me!" he jeered, "and when you get tired of believing all that BS, we can go and have some real fun on a Sunday."

I don't deny wishing I wasn't struggling with cable knit tights and Mary Janes. I wanted to know what the real fun was he was talking about.

This morning he'd pushed Mom's buttons until she got so angry, she slammed cupboards and swore like a sailor, which made him laugh harder and say, "You better get to church and confess that."

Mom screeched out of the driveway, and we took off down the road. She gripped the steering wheel tight in both hands, and the car jerked around a bit like when dad drove, but eventually, by the time we pulled into the parking lot, she had calmed down, and we entered the building resembling a normal church-going family, minus a father.

My sister and I began the morning up with Mom in the sanctuary, but after the first two hymns, Pastor D. called the kids to the front steps of the altar. He situated his robes and sat down with us all crowded around for a children's sermon. He passed around an object lesson and drove some point home, then dismissed us for Sunday School in the basement, while the adults had a sermon, a similar point being driven home but with bigger words and taking much longer.

It was damp and cool in the church basement, with a smell that spoke of long forgotten secrets, whispered from one ear to another, pledged to silence in a dank tomb. Even the lights seemed dim, fighting for breath in this underground cavern. The Presbyterian church basement gave me the creeps.

The clammy air produced goose bumps on my short-sleeved arms as we sat for our morning Sunday school class in a semi-circle of little wooden chairs. My seat was not level, and if I rested back on it, the culprit short leg clunked against the cement floor, echoing louder than an innocent incident like that should. The second time it happened, the teacher looked up and over at me. Not a nasty look or even a warning, but with just a hint of disapproval playing around her eyes, and something deep inside of me desperately wanted to please this woman. To avoid any future noise, I held still with perfect posture, my chilly arms wrapped around my chest.

The teacher sat in the center and smiled both warmly and a little nervously at us. A chunky Bible rested in her lap. She positioned a picture of a young boy in the center of her blue flannel board and held it high so everyone could see. He had dark curls and wore what looked like a bathrobe with leather sandals.

"Children, David was going to be king someday, but he once was little just like you. When he was younger, he was chased by King Saul, who wanted to kill him. David was afraid, and he had to hide in a cave." She added a stone backdrop to the board and placed David in it.

"Hmmm, I wonder if it was a cave like this one?" I thought to myself. "Where's an animal skin when you need one?"

She went on. "When he was afraid, David would pray and sing songs to God." She stuck a harp to the picture, placing it in David's hands.

"Children, do you ever feel afraid?" She asked her leading question and looked around, hoping for some class participation.

"Every hour of every day," I answered silently.

I wanted to raise my hand and tell her, confess to the whole class that when my mother peeled out to take my sister and me to church this morning, her last spitting words to my father were, "Don't be here when we get back."

I was afraid of what would happen if he wasn't. The fight from this morning would likely pick up right where it left off, and that would make for a crap day of my sister and me sitting in our room, listening to them argue.

I felt equally uneasy about him being gone. I was not worried about his daily outings in his van, his trips to Zander's Lake for a hike, or if he whiled away the afternoon, driving randomly on rustic roads. I worried about the permanent exit, if his empty threats of heading to California, once and for all, became a reality. At an almost subconscious level, a part of me wondered how he would survive in the world, out there on his own. Even as a child, I realized and doubted he would make it without us to take care of him.

As these thoughts swirled in my mind and gained intensity, my arm felt as heavy as lead. Somehow, I knew that wasn't the answer she was looking for. A complicated answer like that might escalate the hint of disapproval around her eyes into a frown, or worse yet, an after-class discussion involving parents or preachers.

I kept quiet, and busily picked at a fingernail, until a boy sitting next to me raised his hand and confided that he had been afraid when it thundered last night.

"Excellent!" the teacher beamed.

This was an acceptable answer, and one that could comfortably segue into the solution of praying and singing during thunderstorms.

We rounded out class by standing and singing "Only a Boy Named David", complete with hand motions as the sling went 'round and 'round. The boys cut up and dropped to the floor when the giant came a'tumbling down.

"Praise God from whom all blessings flow!" As the organ and the congregation pealed out the Doxology upstairs, class was dismissed. We emerged from the basement, squinting like raccoons in the brightness of the church lobby.

Parents smiled as they picked up their children, who sported red Kool-Aide moustaches and a coloring picture of King David plucking his harp, both signs of a successful Sunday school session.

We pushed open the heavy double doors and went out into the parking lot, my sister and me tagging along behind our mother. Across town, down the street, and around the corner we drove, to find an empty driveway. My heart pumped as we climbed the stairs and entered the quiet apartment.

I did a quick check. All his important stuff was still here. His prescriptions were on the counter, his coin collection on his desk. Just his thermos and his jacket were gone, so he would be back by sundown. My fears were abated until the next thunderstorm.

CHAPTER 16
Fly Away Home

It was a bright sunny day, a day for wearing shorts and a T-shirt and riding my bicycle. I headed through the tall grass to the backyard shed to get my bike out and found Dad busy at work. He had planks of wood laying in the yard, massive sheets of plastic, a staple gun, and a variety of other tools sprinkled everywhere. Dad had a look of determined concentration on his face and beads of sweat ran down the back of his neck. He had taken off his T-shirt and tied it around his head like a sweatband. I gauged the situation to determine whether it was a good idea to speak.

"What are you doing, Dad?" I asked casually and carefully.

At first there was silence, and I regretted interrupting him, but eventually he grunted and looked up at me.

"Building a glider," he said, wiping his face with the hem

of his T-shirt. "I'm gonna make this baby fly."

I had no idea what to say to that. A part of me was intrigued and proud that Dad was up to something. Another part of me thought "here we go again," another crazy plan, and I worried about the repercussions when his invention didn't work. He would be upset for days, and we would all take the brunt.

Perhaps it was an early symptom of Huntington's disease which caused first one fixation and then another for my dad. According to the HDSA Center of Excellence at the University of Pennsylvania, perseveration and obsessive behavior are common HD behaviors. Those affected can become stuck on an idea, have difficulty switching from one inspiration to another, and become irritated or angry when having to do so. In our house, this was simply how Dad operated. When he had an idea, everything else got dropped until he conquered it or gave up.

Dad was building a hang glider. He had been fascinated with gliders for quite some time now, and when Dad was hooked on something, there was no turning his mind elsewhere. He and his buddy had been planning a trip out to Michigan to try hang gliding at Warren Dunes State Park. At first it seemed like all talk, jaw-flapping dreaming amongst two guys about a road trip and flying like a bird, but now it seemed like it might actually happen.

Dad had it in his mind that he was going to build this hang glider, and they were going to take it with them to Michigan to fly. I can remember being happy that Dad had found a friend since his cousin wasn't around anymore. Dad's new friend was a mail carrier, and when he finished his postal route, he and Dad spent lots of time together, biking the Sugar River State Trail, driving country roads, and talking.

My dad was his friend's sponsor, and while I wasn't completely sure what that meant at the time, it seemed like a grown-up responsibility. I knew what AA was, and even though my dad had beers, he wasn't like the dads on the after-school specials who were Alcoholics. I knew my dad wasn't an Alcoholic, what was wrong with him didn't have a name, unless it was "The Shakes", and I feared that might be worse.

Over the weeks of summer their talk got serious, but Dad was a big dreamer, so I was still skeptical. He came up with so many things that never actually transpired, but if his friend was involved, they might really do this, and I felt both optimistic and relieved. Together, they would drive safely, and his friend could protect him and take care of him. This was much longer than a day trip. Warren Dunes State Park is a coastal dune site along the Lake Michigan coast about 14 miles north of the Indiana border, a half-day drive and three states away. They planned to train at Tower Hill which rises 240 feet above the great lake.

After a few weeks of attempting to make his own hang-glider, Dad packed up his supplies and stowed them in the shed, but instead of giving up entirely in anger, he simply said that they were going to rent gliders from the school, so he didn't need to waste his time building one. Plans for the trip were underway.

A few weeks later, they set out. Mom, my sister, and I waited for updates. There were no cell phones, e-mails, or social media posts, so we simply had to hope that things were going okay. Days went by, and it was weird not having him home. There were parts of me that were afraid he wouldn't come back and others that were equally afraid that he would, with everything turning out as a disaster.

One afternoon, a little over a week since they had left, the van pulled back into the driveway, and the guys climbed out, all grins and smiles and tales of adventure. They had done it, and Dad had the pictures to prove it. He proudly showed photos of him taking lessons, and I still could not believe it. My heart swelled with pride. My chest was so full. Our family feasted on this meal for weeks, the pictures spread out on the coffee table, and Dad visibly strutting around the apartment, reliving the glory.

If he could do this, maybe he was okay? Maybe we would all be okay? I had never heard of a bucket list before, but I now know my dad was filling his. He knew that both his time on this earth and the time remaining for which he would have control of his body was winding down, and he wanted to get a few things in.

CHAPTER 17
King Bathtub

"Magoo! Get in here!"

He called me by the nickname that I hate. I went slowly, dragging my feet to the bathroom door. "Not another one of these marathon lectures from the bath!" I thought to myself.

Since we lived in an older home, with the upper story converted into our apartment space, each room had slanted walls, including the bathroom. You had to crouch down when bathing, and there was no shower stall, in fact, I wasn't aware that people showered in their homes until my first sleep-over at a friend's house in middle school.

My father reigned, and the tub was his throne. Like Tarzan in his loin cloth, he would lie back, hand towel barely draped over his private parts, and often summoned me and required me to sit on the radiator cover and listen. To what?

Anything he considered imperative at the hour. It might have been that the last person who bathed hadn't hung their wet towel up properly or had left the shampoo bottle open. Or, it might be random topics, a collection of what was not right in the world and why it was my fault. Dad often complained about Mom during these bathroom speeches, his voice would rhythm up and down and get faster and faster with agitation. If I complained about privacy or feeling hot or uncomfortable, he would launch into another tirade of "it's just skin", and why was I so uptight like my mother?

The humidity would rise, and perspiration would bead up on my forehead and upper lip. I dared not complain, as this would launch "King Bathtub" into an even longer dissertation on the evil in the world and my lack of intervention. Finally, after what seemed like an eternity, he would release me with, "You can go!" or "Get out of here and let me finish my bath!", as if it had been my idea to visit in the first place. I would waste no time escaping on out of there, the cool breeze of the kitchen air causing shivers on my sweaty arms.

So, it was with trepidation that this day I turned the knob of the old rickety bathroom door. It would not budge. It was locked.

"I can't get in. It's locked," I attempted an excuse.

No luck. I wasn't getting off that easy.

"Jiggle the handle," he ordered.

If we had owned anything of value, our upstairs rental would have been a thief's dream, as "jiggling the handle" was the secret to opening most any of our locked doors. I wiggled the knob back and forth repeatedly and, sure enough, the lock was persuaded, and the door swung open.

I averted my eyes until, by peeking discretely, I could be assured that the hand towel was in place. I then began to scout the area for anything out of place, preparing myself for his anger and how to proactively deescalate it. Medicine cabinet door closed, no laundry on the floor, no water spilled anywhere. I was not prepared for what my eyes met next.

Blood was everywhere. It was streaming down his face and neck, running over his chest, and swirling into delicate patterns which floated on the surface of the bath water. He laid still, eyes closed.

Shocked, I stood riveted and speechless at the doorway. Finally, I cried out, "Dad, Daddy!"

His eyes remained closed, and he gave no response.

"Are you okay?" I whimpered from the spot in which my feet were fixed.

He cracked his eyes to slits and moaned. I began to cry, silently, and when he opened his eyes further and saw the quiet tears slipping down my cheeks, he stirred and sat up. The water sloshed under his weight and drops of blood commingled with the waves.

He smiled a lopsided grin, "I'm okay, I just cut myself shaving."

He gave me a wink. "Hand me another washcloth, will you?"

I yanked clumsily and frantically on the glass knobs of the built-in dresser in our bathroom. The drawers were sticky from years and multiple coats of paint, the humid air, and the lack of a ceiling fan. When I was finally able to wrench it open, I dug in the drawer and passed him a face towel. He began to wipe up the blood, meticulously, one slow swipe at a time, and I waited, rooted in place, and not daring to move.

"Fooled ya, didn't I? You were really worried, weren't you?" he asked.

I blinked.

Serious now, he looked at me intently and asked, "You'd be sad if your 'Old Man' kicked, wouldn't you be?"

I nodded, still not capable of words, and my insides were disjointed and schizophrenic. My heart cried, "Yes, because I would be alone." My head screamed, "No, because you would finally be gone."

"Good, that proves you love me. You can go now." He was at once gruff and aloof.

I turned and ran, the kitchen air cooling the hot tears on my face. Had I passed some sort of test? I certainly did not feel the victor.

CHAPTER 18
Junking

The morning sun shined, not a cloud in the sky, and for once, Dad wasn't sleeping the day away. I ran down the steps of our apartment to find him rummaging around in his van, back doors open and whistling, all good signs.

"Hey Dad," I cautiously peeked in hoping I didn't catch him off guard or change the mood.

"Booper Magoo! Wanna come junkin' with me today?" he asked.

Ugh, I hated that nickname! Wait, did he say, "junking?"

"Sure!" I said, trying not to sound too excited, which might jynx it.

"Well, get in the van then, we don't have all day." He called over his shoulder and grunted as he rearranged tubs and bins in the back.

I piled in the front seat before he closed the back doors, and we were off. Dad tuned the radio and sang along with Steely Dan, something about reeling in years and stowing away time.

"Junking" was Dad's name for doing just that, picking up junk. His route spanned all through Green County, southern Wisconsin, dumpster diving for aluminum cans, steel, and copper wire. Along the way he'd find other treasures, but he was mostly after metal for the recycling center, and on the rarest of days, he invited me to come along.

"I'm my own boss," he'd brag, "Turning people's trash into cash!"

Today was a window down day for both of us, and I stuck my head out, just enough to blow my already messy hair around but not so far to get in trouble. It was all about balance and knowing where the lines were on days like this.

Dad pulled over at all his usual stops, and I waited in my seat while he rummaged through rubbish. It was a good day, and the van was full by noon.

Our last stop was the buyer's garage, run by a huge man with a hairy belly hanging out under his shirt and over his pants like a bottom lip.

"Who's this?" He eyed me slowly and scratched the exposed skin between his shrunken T-shirt and his belt.

"She's my little helper today," Dad said. I was hiding behind him, but at those words, I stepped out and gave a small smile.

"She's going to break some hearts," the owner said.

"No shit," my dad said.

They slapped each other on the back, but then it was down to business, as Dad put his copper on the scale, and they went back and forth about the price of this and that and something about the market. Dad didn't look happy, but he came around, and the man then handed him a stack of bills, which Dad stuffed in his wallet.

The return trip was quiet but not in a scary way, it was calmer, like pressure had been released from a can. Dad left the radio on one station and hummed along to slower songs like "Let Your Love Flow" and "Take it to the Limit", while I leaned my head against the window and dozed off.

When we got home, I announced to my sister, "I went junking with Dad today!"

She rolled her eyes and said, "Good for you, gross."

Her words poked me, but I tried to ignore them and remember the positives. The singing, the breeze blowing, and the proud feeling that Dad did some work today left a warm spot in my stomach where worry usually lived. If every day could be like today, I wondered if our lives would be different? But if every day was like today, would it have been as special?

CHAPTER 19
Christmas on Eggshells

While Elvis Presley lamented his "Blue Christmas", I sat quietly on the living room rug, waiting for my turn to help decorate the tree. The celebration of Christmas at our apartment involved strict protocol, the aligning of stars, and the King of Rock and Roll in equal if not greater proportion to the King of Bethlehem.

Dad, and only Dad, assembled the artificial tree, and it was a Christmas miracle if he didn't launch the branches across the room in frustration before the task was complete. The music on the turntable soothed him, and he would sing along while he worked.

Then came the lights, in a particular and certain arrangement. Finally, Mom got to weigh in, with her favorite blue baubles and a few nostalgic pieces that were fragile, so we couldn't touch. After that, if all was still calm and bright, my sister and I would each get turns to hang ornaments carefully on branches that were at our respective heights, and Mom would snap photos of us doing so. A successful decorating event was rounded out by turning off all the lights in the house except the tree and admiring it from the couch.

When I wasn't focused on the tree, the lights, and whether everyone was getting along, I was wondering whether Dad would come to church with us, even at my age knowing that this held pros and cons either way. Right now, Dad was barefoot and shirtless in sweatpants. After muttering "Christ, it's 100 degrees in here," he had finally coaxed the angel to balance on top of the tree. What would he wear to the service and how irritated would he be after putting it on? According to Dad, clothes were too hot and too tight, choking him so he couldn't breathe.

Mom cleared her throat. "Girls, time to get ready for church," she said, and we popped up like soldiers and got to it, matching dresses already laid out in our room.

At this prompting, Dad rose from his rocking chair and made a move for their own bedroom, which still didn't mean he'd decided to go. My sister and I struggled with our tights and buttoned up each other's backs. After Mom combed the snarls out of my hair while I tried not to yell, I went back out to the living room, and there he was.

Dad wore his darkest pair of blue jeans, and a white

cable-knit sweater. He had combed his hair and feathered it back around his face and glasses. When he slipped on his tan sheepskin coat, I thought he looked handsome, but that he also must be nervous, because he fidgeted like I did when I had to go to the bathroom and had ants in my pants. He jingled his keys in one pocket and loose change in the other and said, "Let's get going."

Mom smiled, and we hurried on down the steps and into the car. Christmas Eve Candlelight service was her favorite, and I could tell it made her happy that Dad was coming along. The Candlelight service was shorter and full of songs, so I somehow knew this would be more bearable for my dad, who usually swore off church sermons as "mumbo jumbo."

The lights were already low, and the organist was going to town on "The First Noel" when we arrived. We slid into a middle pew after a bit of discussion on how close to the front Mom wanted to be versus how close to the back Dad wanted to be. I felt relieved at their compromise. The carols had us up and down in our seats which was fine by Dad, who was shifting, crossing, and re-crossing his legs every minute.

During the message, Dad clasped his hands tightly together and twiddled his thumbs, first one direction, then the other. He was a ball of energy, snorting and clearing his throat, and I grew anxious that other people in our row would notice. Just when it seemed he'd spring out of his seat, the pastor announced it was time for the "Light of the World." Ushers passed each pew distributing candles from baskets, and Pastor instructed that everyone got one, even children, as long as their parents kept an eye out for dripping wax.

I heard the beginning strains of "Silent Night", and the flame was passed from one person to the next, until the entire sanctuary lit up. Dad held his candle in one hand with his other arm wrapped around my shoulder, and as we moved into verse two, his hand shook and melted wax dribbled off the candle wick, down the stem, and onto the circle protector.

I froze in place, and my eyes widened, as the hot liquid traveled, threatening to breach the cardboard, and run down his hand. He must have sensed my fear because his free arm left my shoulder, and he steadied the candle with both hands, holding it like a throttle. In the ultimate irony, a child watched a parent's candle for the remaining chorus and released a held breath when we finally extinguished them and headed for the exit.

As much as Dad detested church, he loved Pastor D., and our family stood in the greeting line before leaving. Pastor D.'s electric smile lit up even bigger when he saw Dad.

"Merry Christmas, my brother! It's so good to see you!" he said and grabbed Dad's hand. They shook in the guy embrace way, hands clasped tight over thumbs and grabbing each other's elbows. They smiled and exchanged words about not being a stranger, and then Pastor D. turned and stooped down eye-level to me with another wide grin.

"Merry Christmas, young lady!"

I was suddenly shy but returned his smile, and we walked out into the chilly night air. If tradition held, we'd drive slowly around neighborhoods looking at the outdoor lights and then eventually head home to open gifts. Santa would have come to fill stockings, although I already knew it had been Mom pretending to forget her purse and going back upstairs to fetch it before we left earlier this evening.

As we wandered through the streets of town, we were quiet and at peace. I looked at the lights and thought about how Pastor D. seemed genuinely happy to see us, my dad especially, and I held onto that hearty handshake like the gift that it was.

CHAPTER 20
Wet Mittens

Those impacted by HD often experience unsolicited irritation and bouts of rage that can last hours and even days, often aimed at their family members and caregivers. Before I knew what likely caused my dad's outbursts, I attempted to prevent them by learning and anticipating his triggers.

According to The National Institute of Health, a common and detrimental neuropsychiatric alteration in those with HD is irritability, which frequently manifests as abrupt and unpredictable outbursts of anger. This anger can be managed with a variety of psychotropic medications or, in the case of my house, by not poking the bear, avoiding landmines, or making yourself very small.

HD irritability is thought to result from the complex relationship between the primary neurobiological changes occurring as the disease progresses and secondary psychological effects. The cognitive decline may be experienced as a kind of overload, which contributes to the irritability. The clinical phenotype of irritability in HD is often reported by family members, as they are usually the patient's primary caregivers and, unfortunately, the common target of the resulting aggression.

An undiagnosed Huntington's disease patient will not be offered medications to ease irritability nor understand why this is happening to them. The undiagnosed patient's family will not report these symptoms to a healthcare professional, rather they will cope and deny and experience shame, certain there is something wrong but unable to put a finger on it.

As my father's HD symptoms began to manifest, he raged, and I became a scholar and a compiler of the "Book of Dad," which contained a thick mental anthology of rules and regulations to avoid pissing him off. The challenging part of these pages was that the content changed with the wind, all depending on his mood. His aggressive episodes or outbursts could be triggered by the slightest aggravation, which would incite angry or violent behavior that lasted for hours to days.

Queue the trigger of wet mittens. In 1979, the winter I turned nine years old, I made the mistake of returning from school with wet mittens in my backpack. On the weekends, when my sister and I came in from playing in the backyard, we placed the wet clothing on the radiator in our shared bedroom. The fabric would sizzle like coals in a sauna, spreading steam and an odor of sweat throughout the room. Depending on the day, this was an acceptable practice, but in just the right temper, if the stars misaligned, I would be in for it. As soon as I got in the door, I scurried to put those drippy mittens on the heat, but I wasn't fast enough.

Dad barged in, already in a foul mood about something. He halted, and his eyes trained on me as I tried to casually arrange the mittens. "What in the hell do you think you're doing?" he thundered.

He began shifting back and forth, always a bad sign, and I could see his mind working as he formulated the words. He threatened to get rid of mittens altogether. If I couldn't be responsible, then I wouldn't have them to wear. My mind fast-forwarded to how that would work at school, what would I say to the teacher and my friends, that I lost them? He looked serious, and I believed him.

No talking back with excuses or explanations, which would only prolong the episode, as my father paced and gestured, his voice rising and falling like a tent revival preacher. There was no escaping. You sat there and took your lumps. Not actual lumps, more figurative, because Dad did not hit. He did hit things, holes in doors, flying objects, broken bits around our little apartment, but he drew the line at people. Why then, was I so terrified?

Tonight, the screaming ended before anything got broken, and he stormed out of my bedroom with parting instructions to not see my face until dinner.

Sometimes I wished he would swing and get it over with, one bruise on an arm peeking out beneath a sleeve. The school counselor, with her beady and ever observant eyes could not help but notice. She'd take a break from "Hey Duso, Come on Out," whisk me away from my ABC After School Special of a life, and we would "do a geographic." In the world of recovery, the expression "doing a geographic" is when people attempt to reboot their life, to escape their problematic environment by changing location. While I was not in recovery, it felt like I needed some sort of reprieve, and I would have moved to Siberia if it meant I could escape my current situation.

In Siberia it would be too cold for mittens to melt, clots of snow clinging to wool for eternity, and no penalty to pay.

CHAPTER 21
Recess

Most playgrounds in 1980's midwestern America sported monkey bars, which by today's standards were surely a safety hazard, but were delicious fun, and my elementary school was no different.

In our school yard, metal tubing formed a rocket shape, and at the top of the jungle gym were four slots, premium seats, requiring a reservation and bought with a hefty price of allegiance. High in the sky we huddled, balancing up top like exotic birds in a cage. We held a bar on each side tightly, hands brushing against one another, whispering secrets, and giggling furiously until the bell rang, forcing us to descend, our palms smelling like money.

In any given recess period, these positions were occupied by the same golden few. There were two Tammy's, one with an 'i,' and a Shelly, but the fact that I can no longer remember their sequence in the lineup is evidence of how their stars paled against the planet for which I orbited, who was Kathy.

Kathy was the Queen of the Fourth Grade and ruled the galaxy of our play gym, determining who sat where and when, what games we played, and the topics covered during our minutes of recess freedom. To the right of the queen was a coveted honor, or to the left a close second. Straight across could be a scary place if she leveled her gaze at you, but any one of those three openings held the lucrative draw of belonging.

If you have done your math, you have already discovered that there would be an odd girl out. Speed was your friend, and when the bell rang, it paid to scoot out there and climb up, not too high in assumption you had already earned a place, but enough to slide in when the nod permitted. Most days Tammy with a 'y' was relegated to the merry-go-round or tetherball, unless one of the others was sick.

In the winter months we would leave our jungle gym thrones for the long metal slide, an equally dangerous apparatus with an open staircase and no guard rails. We hauled armloads of snow up the ladder and then packed the slide with it so we could barrel down like a luge, headfirst until the playground monitor took notice and blew her whistle, and then feetfirst the proper way.

For a reason that only the queen would know, that season her entertainment of choice was trading outerwear, including coats, scarves, and boots. I was petrified. As an avid student and contributing author to the "Book of Dad," and remembering last year's consequences for wet mittens alone, I was quite sure switching snow gear would fall into the category of a high offense. Each recess period I took great care to avoid puddles and not tarry in piles of snow so that my gear dried more easily back home.

But this was the queen of the playground kingdom, and she wanted to wear my snow pants. I have no idea why, they were faded hand me downs from my sister, one zipper that didn't fasten, split alligator teeth running down my left leg. But Kathy's snowsuit was a bright ocean blue puffy one piece. Without thinking further, I stepped in, sliding up the zipper and feeling the down insulation. What could go wrong in thirty minutes?

My stomach wringed knots as Kathy got drenched that day. She flew down the slide and into a pile of mid-day Spring slush, then scaled the ladder and did it again. When the lunch break ended, we peeled everything off in the foyer and switched back. She grabbed her snack and smiled at me while I hung my sad ensemble up on its hook and followed her into the classroom. I heard it dripping on the linoleum from my desk, and I prayed they would dry during reading time.

At the final dismissal, she rode the bus, and I walked home, squishing with each step, and increasing dread. Nearing my street, the crossing guard stopped traffic, and as I crossed I craned my neck around her sign to see if he was home. No blue van in the driveway. "Sweet Hallelujah Jesus!" I thanked the latchkey gods as I ran up the green steps, stripped out of my soggy snow pants, and threw them on the radiator, which let out a hiss and began doing its job.

Time was of the essence, and I contemplated my options. If my sister painted her nails she might draw his fire, as the smell of lacquer held a chapter of its own in the "Book of Dad," with an entire appendix forbidding the use of nail polish, hair spray or perfume. But she did not, instead she sat with a mirror propped up on a pillow, winding her hair into tiny braids all over her head. She would sleep like that and wake up with waves, and she offered to do mine, a rare moment of generosity, but I was too nervous to accept.

"No thanks," I said.

"Suit yourself," she said and laid back on her bed, opening *Teen Beat* magazine.

I watched the clock. It had been a warm day, but the March sun still set early in the Midwest, and it would not be long now. My best chance was to have every other upsetting variable taken care of before Dad's return. Daylight Savings Time saved me, buying an extra hour, and by the time the blue van pulled in, I had finished my homework, ate a PBJ and was innocently reading a book in our room.

I heard him scale the outside steps, then enter through the porch, and drop his keys and other contents of his pockets on the kitchen counter. Dad lumbered into our bedroom, never knocking or considering privacy. I kept silent as he surveyed the area, eyeing for anything out of place and breathing noisily, clearing his throat, and fidgeting with his glasses.

"Did you eat?" he broke the silence and asked.

"Yes," my sister and I said in unison.

He ran his hand across the radiator, briefly patted the damp snow pants and mittens, hmphed, and left without another word. I heard the TV switch on and the familiar theme song of *Three's Company* inviting us to knock on their door because they had been waiting for us. Canned laughter filled the air.

I had been granted a stay, and I let out the breath I'd been holding for what seemed hours. I had survived another day of recess in the fourth grade, and managed to appear normal to my friends, but it was becoming increasingly clear to me that there weren't enough pages in the "Book of Dad" to handle all situations that might be coming my way.

CHAPTER 22
A Dash of Sugar

The Mayo Clinic cites depression as the most common psychiatric disorder associated with Huntington's disease, followed by irritability, sadness or apathy, social withdrawal, insomnia, loss of energy and frequent thoughts of suicide. Other common psychiatric disorders that carpool with HD are obsessive-compulsive disorder, manic spells, and bipolar, a condition with alternating episodes of depression and mania.

My dad had no shortage of the items on this list, and as his symptoms began to reveal themselves in his early 30's, he was affected with bipolar tendencies, seasons of dark and light. He had yet to be diagnosed, so our family navigated this mysterious landscape, the ebb and flow of his moods, and held on to any substance of convention, which could sometimes be found in the kitchen.

With a look of serious determination on his face and a steady pulse of internal energy, Dad's intensity measured equally against the pleasure he took in cooking. He was happy and purposeful in the kitchen.

I knew he was up to something when I discovered all the cookware we owned spread on the counter. He tucked a dish towel in the band of his underwear and tossed another over his bare shoulder, using them to wipe his hands or make dramatic swipes at sweat beading on his face. His long, unkempt hair combed back, glasses pushed higher than usual on his nose, Dad was all business. We hadn't had a hot meal in days, and I dared hope today he wouldn't crash in the middle.

Dad was making American Goulash, and it smelled like heaven, ground beef sizzled in one pan, tomatoes in another, and pasta boiled in one more. Dad obsessively stirred the sauce, lifting the lid, sampling, analyzing. I desperately wanted to stay, willing myself invisible so as not to be unceremoniously booted from the kitchen. I felt proud of my dad, who produced amazing dishes out of whatever he pulled from the refrigerator, provided the mood was right.

In this rare moment of emulation, I leaned against the wall by the stove, nibbling from a box of Cracker Jack and studying him carefully. I chewed each sweet piece of popcorn slowly to make it last. Dad glanced over, and I froze.

"That shit is garbage! I could make it from scratch, and it would melt in your mouth!" he snorted.

I remembered that, before I was born, Dad held a short-lived job as a bakery chef. He made caramel corn, gingerbread, and stirred vats of chocolate for a local company which sent out cheese, dobash cake and gift baskets at the holidays. He considered himself not only a connoisseur of sweets, but a specialist in savory dishes as well. He returned his focus to the stove, and I exhaled slowly.

"Always add a dash of sugar to your Goulash," he instructed the air around me, as he sprinkled a tablespoon of the final ingredient in his masterpiece. "It cuts the acid in the tomatoes."

I drank in this puzzling advice, pretending he said it specifically for my benefit, but I doubt he remembered I was there. Dad usually fizzled at clean up, and today was no different. After one last taste test, he retreated to the living room, clicked on the television, and sank into the couch. To keep the peace, I scrubbed the pans and utensils left lying everywhere before Mom got home from her shift.

Dishes done and waiting for the casserole to simmer, I dug for the prize at the bottom of my empty Cracker Jack box. It was never anything much, a tattoo or a sticker, but the anticipation held the hope. This time it was a bright pink plastic ring with a fake diamond, which I forced over a sticky knuckle.

Despite Dad's claims at superior caramel corn, he never made any in our kitchen, but that was okay. Tonight, there was dinner, and I would rest in this calm, before the next storm of emotion or valley of sadness must be weathered. It would be dark for days and then, there would be pots and pans again, and Dad would be cooking. The anticipation held the hope.

CHAPTER 23
Frontal Behaviors and Inhibitions Lost

A book worm from the time I learned my letters, I spent most of my growing up years with my nose buried in one. Books were an escape and a vehicle to other worlds, and they offered hope for alternate endings.

I rode my bicycle to the public library at least once a week and loaded up on a stack that would barely fit in my backpack, then pedaled back home, and devoured them one by one. On summer days, I spent most of my afternoons at the library, enjoying the air-conditioning and the quiet until closing hours, the smell of books and floor wax, endless stacks enclosing me like an embrace.

If my sister was out and Mom was working the PM shift, that left Dad and me to get through an evening together. Once he was in for the night, he paced and watched TV. I typically kept a low profile in my bedroom, but sometimes I ventured out and curled up in Mom's reading chair with my latest book. If Dad was in a foul mood, he wouldn't allow any lamps on in the living room, but otherwise, I could rock there and read, and he didn't mind my company.

"Damn it, it's an oven in here!" Dad said.

Dad couldn't tolerate the heat, or at least that's what he claimed, when he routinely stripped down as soon as he walked in the door each day. My dad was characterized by not wearing a stitch of clothing in the house, and if anyone complained, he'd launch into a long lecture about it being "just skin," so I knew better than to say anything.

Tonight, he laid on the couch, with nothing but a thin blanket covering him. The TV was on low volume, and I kept my eyes on my book. Dad couldn't get settled, and although I was used to him fidgeting, tossing, and turning, tonight felt different and wrong. He flapped the covers repeatedly, and I raised my eyes over the pages and saw rhythmic movement, increasing in speed. I didn't fully understand what was happening, and although he appeared completely unaware of my presence, I was frozen and didn't dare move or bring attention to myself. Doesn't he know I am sitting right here? I fixed my eyes onto the page, willing them to soften, and mentally fled the scene. Soon all was quiet except for his snores, and I quietly exited the room.

The frontal lobes of the brain are crucial for decision-making, impulse control, and social behavior. As HD progresses, these lobes slowly deteriorate, and this can lead to significant changes in personality called frontal behaviors or even Frontotemporal Dementia (FTD.) FTD with a behavioral variant (bvFTD) is most known for loss of inhibition.

The Mayo Clinic sites bvFTD symptoms which include inappropriate social behavior, loss of empathy, lack of judgement, repetitive compulsive behaviors, and a loss of inhibitions, including sexual promiscuity or inappropriate sexual behavior.

The National Library of Medicine adds executive dysfunction, the inability to manage a person's own thoughts, and disinhibition, the inability to withhold inappropriate or unwanted behavior, as common psychological symptoms of HD.

Understanding Behavior in Huntington's Disease: A Guide for Professionals by Arik C. Johnson, PsyD and Jane S. Paulsen, PhD, explains that inappropriate sexual behavior and disinhibition is thought to be caused by damage to the caudate nucleus, a deep area of the brain that controls behavior.

In 1980, there was no clipboard with these big words on it, no medical jargon, or scientific studies to explain a father's bizarre behavior to a 10-year-old girl, but my sixth sense told me to pretend it never happened. As I grew older, I became disgusted with his recurring nakedness and frequent inappropriate behavior, but I rarely lashed out, preferring to disappear instead.

CHAPTER 24
A Mutual Habit

"I will never hit you," my father said, twisting the dish towel in his hands, and then his eyes went off to the right of my shoulder. I almost turned around to see what he was looking at, but then I recognized the absent gaze of a mind traveling far away. I could tell a story was coming, and for that I was hesitantly grateful.

For the last thirty minutes I had endured a loud lecture on the correct way to dry dishes because Dad found one still wet in the cabinet. He ordered me to take all the dishes back out of the cupboard and re-dry them one by one while he paced back and forth in the kitchen, opening the refrigerator door and closing it, turning the lights on and off, his voice growing faster and more enraged with each minute.

My hands were shaking, and I was afraid that I might drop a dish. Then there would be no salvaging the rest of the day.

I held the last plate tightly in both hands and used my nose to work my glasses back up where they belonged. It was one of my many nervous habits, the one which Mom was always telling me to stop doing, and the only thing my dad ever told her to leave me alone about.

He began in a quieter and calmer voice. "I used to wrinkle my nose to push up my glasses just like you're doing right now. I felt like my face had to wiggle. Hard as I would try not to do it, it only made it worse. The 'Old Man' hated it when I scrunched up my nose, especially if he was drinking a cocktail in his after-work chair."

Dad described Grandpa with decades of residual bitterness hovering in his eyes and mixed with his voice. How he'd still be in his coveralls, hat resting on his knee, knocking back the first of several drinks quickly, as fast as my grandmother could bring them, then slowing down and sipping the last few, while they worked their magic on his tired body. When Grandpa wanted a refill, he jiggled the empty glass, ice cubes rattling to get her attention.

"If the 'Old Man' was relaxed enough, he might not notice, but usually he started in on me before the second drink hit his system. That night it came out of nowhere," Dad said.

"'Stop that God damn fidgeting!' The work boot was off his right foot in a split second and sailed across the room in my direction. He was dead on, and the heel of that boot hit me square in the eye, shattered my glasses and set my nose to bleeding." Dad paused and took a deep breath.

"So, you see when you're moving your nose or your face, I'm not gonna give you a hard time about it. If you have 'The Shakes' like 'Bean,' and probably me, it could be bad, but that might not happen. If we get it, it won't be until later, so you don't have nothin' to worry about right now. You just enjoy being young."

After that string of compressed words, the silence following them hung heavy in the air.

I knew "Bean," or "String Bean" was my Dad's nickname for his Aunt LuAnne, my Grandma's sister who lived in a nursing home, but I still didn't know exactly what "The Shakes" were, and it didn't sound good. I resented being lumped in with "Bean" just for pushing up my glasses when my hands were full, but I wasn't about to argue.

When he stopped speaking, I waited for his eyes to re-focus and for either the tirade to resume or the freedom of release. After a few minutes, it became apparent that he was to remain lost in thought indefinitely, so I slipped out unnoticed.

I glanced back and saw him there, the dish towel that moments before he had been wringing the life out of, now hung loose and limp in one hand. Dad looked lost in memory, but then just as quickly as he snapped, he sealed back up.

Do fathers feel sad and scared but keep it on the inside?

Do they fold their cracks inward to go on living? Perhaps that is why you see anger on their outer shell, it is protecting the inner rift. I felt the smallest bit of empathy for him, and then, just as quickly, it was gone.

Adult HD symptoms usually start between 30 and 50 years of age and continue to get worse throughout the remainder of the person's life, while Juvenile HD manifests with slowness, stiffness, and muscle twitching comparable to Parkinson's disease.

It is unlikely that either form of Huntington's disease was to blame for the nervous facial tics of a small boy in a stressful home, but his behavior being compared to mine would haunt me. Throughout my early adolescent and adult years, I carried constant paranoia that I would become like my father.

CHAPTER 25
Thanksgiving and Easter Smell Like Cow Pies

Most of the holidays that I remember were celebrated at my Great Uncle and Aunt's farm in southern Wisconsin. These events were noisy, full of good food, and freedom. It always felt like I had fallen through a rabbit hole as we pulled into their gravel drive, and as we rolled past those silos filled with feed, the barbed wire fencing, and enormous mounds of manure, I was reminded how much these sights and smells were foreign compared to my life in a small town, but a city, nonetheless.

We exited the car, and I was greeted by at least a half dozen barn cats, which purred and circled my legs as my mother hurried us toward the house, hissing, "Don't touch those cats, they have diseases!"

My older sister began sneezing as soon as the car door opened.

My great-uncle was a quiet wiry man, but strong as steel. I had no concept of the many chores he already accomplished before I arrived in my itchy Sunday dress, I only remember that he napped after lunch and then quietly slipped out the door to the barn again later that day.

Great Aunt May compensated for his quietness, as she was animated and boisterous, wore a huge smile, and carried her voice many yards. She held court in the kitchen, pulling massive casseroles out of the oven, slicing ham, and swatting flies all at the same time. Barking orders at her two daughters, eventually a table that could hold over twenty people was set to heaving with steaming dishes.

The commotion reached a deafening decibel as relatives poured in the door, carrying pies or slinging suitcases if they were staying over. Family members were everywhere, arguing and cursing, laughing, and hugging each other. I would feel a little sick to my stomach, because at my house, shouting always preceded something unpleasant, but here, it was simply part of the camaraderie.

I also didn't like being put on display, but as each relation entered, they would analyze my vertical inches gained as my mother listed off my latest accomplishments in a couple summary paragraphs. "Yes, she's eleven now, won the school spelling bee, might start babysitting soon."

"Yeesh, get me out of here," I thought to myself, "If a

training bra is mentioned, I will hitch-hike home, I swear."

"Come and get it!"

No dinner bell was required, as everyone heard Aunt May calling and filed to the table. My claustrophobia quite possibly has its roots from this very table. You pulled out your chair, slid into it, and committed to remaining for the duration of the meal. Bathroom breaks? Forget about it, but the smell was intoxicating, a spread of ham, mashed potatoes and green beans, real butter and a million desserts. I tried not to focus on the flies parked everywhere, it happens at picnics, right?

The job of grace was delegated to the oldest nephew, who said the familiar but nonsensical words that always came before a meal at this staunchly Catholic household, followed by mumbles and crossings from the crowd. As the serving platters and bowls were passed around, you had to take now whatever you might conceivably want later, because after that dish went by, it was unlikely to return.

There was a separate small card table set up in the kitchen for Great Uncle Teddy. Why did Teddy get to stretch out in a seat all to himself? Because Teddy had Down's Syndrome, which resulted in some nasty table manners, and I guess no one wanted to sit by him. On occasion, I considered that the extra breathing room might have been worth the risk of catching his syndrome, but Teddy scared me. He looked harmless enough, tooling around in his striped suspenders and black orthopedics, never found without his harmonica in his front shirt pocket. What threw me off the most were his eyes, which must have been the bluest blue when he was younger, but cataracts had clouded them over in ghostly white. Every time I saw Teddy, he asked me to marry him. As I grew older, I often felt sorry that Teddy ate by himself, but the whole proposing thing outweighed my empathy.

If I sat by Grandma, she would pile a big scoop of whatever salad she brought onto my plate. She made a variety of these salads, but they all contained the same basic ingredients in a concoction of canned fruit, Jello, cottage cheese, and Kool Whip. The puffy stuff masqueraded as a dessert, until you took a bite and suddenly little chunks of cottage cheese cropped up everywhere in your mouth. Of all the dishes that might come back around for a second visit, would it be dinner rolls or freshly husked corn? No, it would be the puffy stuff, and if I had managed the "push it around and poke it with your fork" scam with what I'd already been given, sure thing I'd wind up with seconds.

After everyone had eaten their fill, the extrication process began, with the thinnest relatives sliding out first, skinny aunts who headed for the kitchen to rinse plates. Then, children who received the "can I go now?" blessing from parents would slip out next. Those folks with the most around the middle would remain, scooping a little extra onto their plates and kicking back, enjoying the elbowroom.

The escape from that table signaled the beginning of an entire day of release. The aunts were wiping the dishes as if their very lives depended on it. The men all shuffled to the living room to recline in La-Z-Boys and tell stories or fall asleep, and us kids? Well, we were free as birds.

In the winter we explored every nook and cranny of that old farmhouse, with marathon games of hide and seek. My second cousins had cool toys like walkie-talkies and remote-controlled cars, but usually a shortage of batteries, or the toys themselves were broken. I didn't understand that concept since breaking things was not allowed in my house. Just holding a toy that had seen better days caused me to look around a little, making sure no one decided to blame me for the mishap.

In mild weather, we went outside and roamed as far as the fence line where the angry bull would snort, challenging, "Come on, make my day!" Then, we'd stroll down through the rows of beans in the garden. Bea would pick them off the vine and eat them raw, but they tasted awful to me that way. I wanted to be like her, so I'd chew them a bit and then spit them out when she wasn't looking. If the weather held out and the parents had good conversations, we might get a stay of at least twilight before someone hollered at us to come in. We would trudge back with dragging feet, the boy cousins heading to the barn to do chores. It felt so good to be forgotten.

In the early years, when Dad still came along with us to

the farm, I would pray that he wouldn't have words with Grandpa and was enjoying himself, so we could stay longer. Drinks would be flowing freely by then and a hot game of cards going on at the freshly cleared table. My Great Aunt Harriet could card shark with the best of them. With long fingernails painted fire engine red, she'd slap her winning hand down triumphantly, while everyone else moaned at their misfortune. She'd chain-smoke and ignore my grandpa while he lectured her on the perils of lung cancer.

If it got much later, Great Aunt May would begin re-heating leftovers from the noon meal. In the best of circumstances, someone would haul out the screen and projector to share vacation slides of Switzerland and other European travels.

I would lay on the shag carpet of their family room, watching the screen but also gazing at my favorite picture on the wall. In a collage of black and white graduation portraits were the five sisters, framed from oldest to youngest: Harriet, Grandma, Eilene, Luanne, and May. They looked like glamorous movie stars, with fur stoles gracing their bare shoulders and their hair done in pin up curls.

Great Uncle Teddy was not in the lineup, but I guessed it was because he didn't graduate. Great Aunt Eilene and her family seldom traveled back from Colorado for holidays. I had never seen Great Aunt Luanne, who everyone here at the farm also called "String Bean," at these family gatherings. I knew that she lived at the nursing home in town because she was sick, but that was all that anyone would say about it.

The equation I put together in my young mind at these holidays was the more drinks, the more fun the big people became, especially my dad. Why, in this rowdy group of relatives, he seemed almost normal! I could breathe here, my dad was just like everyone else, smiling and tipping a few back.

Eventually the evening wound down, and we would head for the car. Mom would argue that she should drive, but Dad would growl "I'm fine!", while climbing into the driver's seat. We'd fly over the hills through the dark, and I'd hear Dad fishing with his foot for the floor high beam controller and concentrating with both hands on the wheel.

I would have eaten Grandma's puffy salad every day if those holidays could have lasted forever.

CHAPTER 26
Sea Legs at High Altitude

Dad and Mom got the travel bug at least once a year, but I remember very little of any of these trips. How could my dad, who drove haphazardly, was easily angered by other drivers, and u-turned at the least provocation, make it through these cross-country road trips? I think the cure for extended time on the road was for him to drive at night while there was less traffic and we all slept, for I remember falling asleep in snow and waking up to palm trees and sunshine on more than one occasion. Then, having to sit still with my sister and be quiet in the hotel room while Dad slept off the drive.

I recall an ocean which tasted terrible, with waves that sucked me in and soaked my shorts before we ate at a restaurant. We once went to an amusement park that had a killer whale in a tank which did tricks for treats. Dad did not seem impressed, perhaps he was thinking, "Get me up there, and I'll make that guy really perform!"

What I do remember with clarity is our annual trips to Colorado to visit Dad's Aunt Eilene, his uncle, and their son, my father's cousin and childhood friend. Each summer we based out of their house and made day trips to Estes Park, exploring the mountains. Dad would purposefully drive too close to the edge of cliffs and take hairpin switchback curves at reckless speed, while Mom held on for dear life. He'd stand on top of lookouts, taking in the view and holding us high in the air with Mom hollering at him to be careful. No trip was complete without Dad pointing out wildlife, such as mule deer or bighorn sheep, and taming the Colorado chipmunks, holding out peanuts and coaxing them until they were eating from his hand.

When I rubbed sleep out of my eyes on these trips I was greeted by the Rocky Mountains, their snowy caps appearing close enough to touch, yet still miles away. My sister and I would color in our books and hold our bathroom needs until we got there. The best part of staying at our relatives' house was that Dad could go sleep off the drive, and we got to get out and play.

I loved going to visit Great Aunt Eilene. Eilene let us pet their hound dog and made us snacks anytime we were hungry. Aunt Eilene looked just like Grandma but skinnier and was always hugging me and smoothing my hair. She raised her eyebrows a lot and wore the same smile as Grandma, which was friendly but a little too wide and appeared drawn onto her face with a marker, which sometimes scared me a little.

We now know that HD can result in upper facial chorea, and the grimace of my great aunt and grandmother was an early indicator of the disease. George Huntington in *On Chorea*, describes facial chorea in the disorder that bears his name as, "the eyelids are kept winking, the brows are corrugated, and then elevated, the nose is screwed first to the one side and to the other, and the mouth is drawn in various directions."

On this visit, something was especially off. We arrived just before dinner, and I could tell right away that something was wrong. Eilene's smile was wider than ever, and she shrugged her shoulders in what appeared constant uncertainty. As we finished eating, she got up to clear the plates, and I came to the startling realization. She walked like my dad.

Anxiously, I watched Great Aunt Eilene carry a platter across her kitchen. That plate bobbled and weaved up and down like the flight of the bumblebee, and it appeared at any moment, as if it would come crashing to the kitchen tile. The thought of things breaking, especially glassware, sent shivers down my spine, as broken things usually meant for a bad day at my house. Just as I was about to develop a quiet ulcer, the plate found a home on the counter. Whew. Then, off she went with a dishtowel, drying a drinking glass and holding several others in the crook of her arm! Would this never end?

She traveled with a slightly tilted gait, a hop-step. She smiled and mumbled to herself the entire time she cleaned up after our evening meal, her head swaying with a mind of its own, her words nonsensical.

This was the first summer we had come to Colorado and found her obviously symptomatic. Earlier that year I had heard through the parental eavesdrop line that she was sick. I was sure it was the secret disease in our family that the grownups spoke of in hushed tones around the farm table when the children were supposedly playing. I wondered if they whispered because they thought we had it too and didn't want to wreck our lives by telling us early.

I had heard them say that there was no cure, and I wondered if they could tell by looking at you whether you had it or not, because they would whisper with each other while looking up and around at us cousins. Their eyes would fix on one of us, and they would be shaking their heads as if to say, "Oh, yes, that one there, she's in for it. Should we tell her now? No, let's wait a few years, let her enjoy her childhood."

I sat frozen in my seat while my great aunt finished, alternating between chewing my fingernails and wondering whether I should offer to help. With clean up finally done, my sister and I were excused to run outside, where I promptly climbed the tree in their side yard and tuned my little transistor radio. Static came through, and then Anne Murray crooned about finding a little hideaway. I didn't know exactly what the song meant, but I closed my eyes and held it to my ear, allowing the music to soothe me, equally desperate for a refuge.

When our week-long visit ended, the car was packed, and I wanted to hug my Great Aunt Eilene goodbye, but I was terrified of whatever had taken over her body. I was afraid she might uncontrollably grab me, or tip over, and it would be my fault. Most of all, I was afraid I would catch what she had if I got too close. I hopped in the car with a quick wave and downcast eyes.

Hours down the road, I wished I could have gone back and held her tight. I was proud of her, forging through the kitchen like nothing, not even a bad case of sea legs, would stop her from getting the dishes done. She had a lot of guts.

How many times are we paralyzed by our present circumstances, imagining the what ifs, and dwelling on hypotheticals. Great Aunt Eilene was a lesson to me in doing the next logical thing in the face of an uncertain future.

CHAPTER 27
Lifted Grounding

Because Great Aunt Eilene and her family had moved to Colorado, they didn't usually make the long trip to Wisconsin for gatherings, so the holiday that she came home to the farm, there was something in the air. Even the young have antennae, and I suspected she had gotten worse, and feared that it must be "The Shakes."

This year the normally festive mood was subdued, conversations were hushed, and Eilene kept to the back room, like a secret. Only a few people went in at a time to see her. She took her meal on a TV tray, and I took that to mean she didn't want people to watch her eat, or like Uncle Teddy at the card table, maybe the family didn't want to watch her eat.

After I had been excused from the big table, I asked my mom if I could go back and see her. Dad and Mom gave me a surprised look, then their eyes connected above my head for a silent but visual vote. In unison they nodded and let me go.

I sat on the floor at her feet, careful not to disrupt her tray. She was wearing a soiled bib, and Great Aunt May was clearing her plate and wiping her face like a child. I had a moment of panic when I wanted to bolt, but something kept me there, and then it was pretty much like old times.

I did the talking because she couldn't really communicate. I told her all about school and the stuff I was up to. She smiled, ear to ear, but it was that exaggerated combination of grin and grimace. She kept nodding her head and repeating the same phrase over and over, her words garbled like she had a mouth guard in. Her thin arms waved, and her forefingers touched her thumbs like she was making shadow puppets.

What I remember most about this visit happened on the way home. Earlier in the week I had been grounded for something, surely some minor infraction from the "Book of Dad," and had been kept indoors for days, no playing with friends, no riding my bike, no trips to the library. As we drove home that night, Dad adjusted the radio volume down and cleared his throat.

"What you did tonight, seeing 'Leeney' for a bit, that was good." He paused and cleared his throat again.

"We're proud of you, and your mom and I are lifting your grounding."

"Okay," I said flatly, and kept my eyes trained out the window.

They had reduced my sentence. I wondered at the time what I had done so special to get the punishment lightened. Was Great Aunt Eilene that scary? That people should be rewarded for spending time with her? I wanted to ask if I could have caught "It" by being too close to her, but I didn't think they would have let me go back there if this disease was that kind of contagious.

This sickness surrounded our family, and I had gathered but bits and pieces from overheard conversations. If Dad shuffled and shrugged like Eilene, did he have it too? If I wrinkled my nose, did I? If "The Shakes" came to our house, would people need rewards to come and see me?

CHAPTER 28
Allowances, Nickels, and Skipping Lunch

In middle school I was flat-chested, awkward and wore thick glasses. I had a circle of friends who seemed to all have nicer clothes, newer bikes, and plenty of spending money. For all the family trips we went on, we never had any money for designer clothes or Nike tennis shoes, and I found myself scrapping for every spare bit of cash I could come by to keep pace with my group.

My sister and I both received a weekly allowance of five dollars in exchange for doing chores, and Mom would hand it over each week when she got paid. Dad also got an allowance, and Mom would place it on the kitchen table, two crisp twenty-dollar bills still in the First National Bank envelope.

How she set Dad's allowance on the table depended on her mood. If it was a good day, she'd set it down normal, but if Dad had been irritating her, she'd set the envelope down harder.

If they had been in the middle of a fight, she'd slam the bills down with words like, "maybe you should get a job."

How Dad picked up his allowance depended on how it had been laid down. Sometimes he was subtle and slipped the twenties into his wallet with one coordinated movement. Other times he was indignant and snatched them up with a big speech about how much he had accomplished lately to earn it, and then argued that he deserved a raise. The worst way, which made my stomach hurt, was when he slid them off the table in shame, tucked them in his pocket, and left the house without a word.

Each payday brought a conflict of emotions. Dad receiving an allowance and not having a real job made me embarrassed and ashamed, but mostly I was irritated that he got so much more than me. I was doing all the chores, while he was driving around in his van and watching baseball games.

Our family income was low enough that we qualified for the public-school system's reduced lunch program. For forty cents I could purchase a hot lunch in the cafeteria. Kids paying regular price paid ninety-five cents for their meal. I was embarrassed to be on reduced lunch. It wouldn't have been so bad if it wouldn't have been so obvious.

First, you had to announce "reduced" when you went through the beginning of the line so the cafeteria lady would know how much to charge you. Then, as you stood in line to pay, every other kid had a dollar. They would snap them, fold them, and whip each other with them. I held my coins in my hand. Each child got a nickel in change, which they plopped on their tray as if it meant nothing and went to find a seat. I had no nickel on my tray. After they were done eating, the kids would play with their nickels. They would spin them, stack them, and throw them at each other. I had no nickel to toss around and found myself eyeing other coins that had fallen to the floor with no one noticing or caring, wondering if it would be too obvious if I scooped them up.

After school, most of us walked by the 19th Street candy store on the way home. For a nickel you could get a Lollipop or a piece of licorice. They would ask me why I wasn't getting anything.

How badly I wanted a nickel! How badly I wanted to fit in! Sometimes Mom had given me two quarters, for which I received a dime in change; other times I had a dollar, which I could wave around with the best of them in line, but then got sixty cents back in change, and once again, no nickel. There was no increment that produced a nickel in change, and any money that I did get back was to be saved for the next day, certainly not pitched around, or wasted on candy.

In hindsight, a child doesn't understand the big picture. What I overlooked was my mom, working overtime to pay our bills. If you take ninety-five cents minus forty cents, that is a daily savings of fifty-five cents or $1.10 for my sister and me. Multiply that by five days a week for over 30 weeks of the term, and it comes to almost $175.00 over the course of a typical school year. $175.00 in 1982 would have bought all my sister's and my school clothes for the year. I wanted those nickels to fit in with my classmates, but they amounted to a significant savings for our family. I should have been grateful, but instead became even more monetarily motivated.

I discovered a plan for augmenting my meager allowance in the form of skipping lunch. It started with a few of the cooler girls at our table who claimed not to be hungry and opted out of the lunch line to sit together sipping on cola purchased from the vending machine. The cans of soda in the machine cost more than my reduced rate, so as I began to sit with them, I went a step further and said I wasn't hungry and wasn't thirsty either.

This scheme went well for several days, and doing the math, I calculated that, if I could continue skipping lunch and pocketing the money, I would easily have enough for the matinee on Saturdays as well as keep banking for the pair of Guess jeans I had my eye on at the shop downtown. I was not prepared for how much my stomach would growl in fifth period! Each afternoon I could barely concentrate on classes and counted the hours until dismissal, praying for my dad to be gone so I could fix a snack once I got home.

I did not anticipate the intervention of a well-meaning lunchroom monitor. Each day Mrs. L. made the rounds, and she was vicious, forcing the boys to pick up dropped food and use their napkins to wipe spilled milk. Her hawk eyes roved the room, detecting any sort of mischief and putting a preemptive stop to it, so it didn't take too many days of our circle skipping lunch before we caught her attention.

"What's going on here girls, why aren't you eating?" she asked, strolling by our table.

We all looked down awkwardly, and eventually the bravest of the group mumbled that we weren't hungry. She paused for the longest time, eyeing each of us and for some reason held my gaze the longest.

"Does your mother know you're skipping meals?" she asked, looking right at me.

"Yes," I said, straightening my posture.

"So, if I called her on the telephone after this and asked her, she'd be alright with it?" She asked, her eyes boring into me.

"Yes, but she works at night, so she might be sleeping and not answer," I said, hoping to discourage her.

"Okay, then I'm going to contact her, and we'll just see."

Mrs. L. turned and strode off purposefully. The other girls rolled their eyes and laughed, saying I put that teacher in her place, but I felt like there was lead in my stomach, and for once in the afternoon, no hunger pains hit me, as my appetite was gone.

The walk home that afternoon was eternal, and the wait for Mom to return from work even longer. I sat out on "The Green," with a book instead of a stuffed animal, but still feeling like a little kid. The hours ticked by, and finally shortly after 11:00 PM she pulled in and climbed the stairs. I tried to see her expression before she opened the screen door. Had Mrs. L. called her at work?

"What are you still doing up?" she asked.

"Oh, I just wanted to say hi to you," I said casually.

She smiled, put her bags down and pulled off her jacket.

"Let me guess, you want a snack?" she asked.

"When don't I?" I answered with a hopeful smile.

We both laughed and went into the kitchen. Dad was watching *Taxi* on TV and didn't come out to interrupt, so we kept our voices down and talked about our days over cold cereal. I mentioned everything but the run-in with the lunchroom monitor and my skipping lunches.

Afterwards, I laid in bed feeling both relieved and guilty. Obviously, Mrs. L. hadn't contacted her, but I couldn't hope it was an empty threat, and she was just trying to scare us. She might call again another night, and it also didn't feel right, taking Mom's money. I decided to go back to my reduced lunch and find another way to earn extra money to fit in.

CHAPTER 29
Babysitting and Other People's Fathers

My sister was now old enough to babysit, and for the past couple years she enjoyed a steady income from all the families at church, while I was considered too young. But before too long, she took her first paying job at a pizza palace, got a steady boyfriend, and became much less available.

One Saturday evening, due to a stroke of her misfortunate forgetfulness and my good luck, a family came to pick up my sister for their date night, and she wasn't home. In a moment of panic, my mother thought to let me go instead and went outside to explain and offer the option to the father parked in the driveway. Within a matter of minutes, the swap was made, and I was buckling my seatbelt, on my way to my first paying gig as a babysitter.

I began minding other people's children every free minute I had, storing away and then blowing my earnings on all the things my friends so casually purchased. Dad would grumble when he saw me count my cash and checks, saying "look at you, making more than your 'Old Man'," but I didn't feel sorry for him. Why didn't he have a real job, like other fathers? These dads who picked me up and drove me to their houses to watch their children while they took their wives out to dinner and the movies, they were nothing like him.

I detected how very different our family was from every other family I encountered while babysitting. I watched these people parent and observed how the children weren't afraid of anything. If they spilled their drink, the mother would simply wipe it up without any yelling or fuss.

In the summer months I had one regular job with a family for which I not only watched the children but also cooked and cleaned. This wasn't my favorite booking because they didn't pay as well, and I had to ride my bike there, clear across town and back, but it was a steady option, and I needed the money. I was saving for a new bicycle with ten speeds.

The final week of the job was the last week of August, and it had been especially grueling, as the mother was expecting another child and had a lengthy list of chores for me each day. In addition to watching her children at swimming lessons and making them lunch, I helped her clear out a baby room, washed mounds of laundry, and scrubbed each bathroom spotless. At the end of the Friday shift, I was not looking forward to the bike ride home, but I was anticipating the paycheck.

"It isn't as much as you were maybe hoping," she said with a small smile and a nervous laugh. "Maybe you can call it a gift to the new baby?"

She handed me some folded bills, and when I glanced at them and did quick math, my heart dropped. This wasn't even as meager as I thought it might be, it was worse. I nodded at her, pocketed the money, and climbed on my old three-speed bicycle, resigned that it would be a much longer time before I could replace it.

I pedaled home with sweat dripping in my eyes and tried not to cry as I felt the salt and sting. I was furious at how hard I had worked for how little I had been compensated, and I was humiliated that I hadn't been brave enough to object. As I stood on the pedals to pump up the hill to our house, I saw my dad's van in the driveway and winced. Why did he have to be home, today of all days? When I didn't want to talk about this, hear any kind of a lecture about breaking another of his stupid rules, and wanted nothing more than peace and quiet and a cold drink from the refrigerator.

I discreetly entered the house. Every curtain was closed to keep out the summer sun, and Dad was pacing in the kitchen in his underwear, his hair a mess. This was never a good sign, but he took one look at my bedraggled state and knew something was wrong.

"What happened?" he asked, eyes intent on my beet red face.

And it all spilled out.

How hard I had worked, how small the pay was, how blasted hot it was outside. My head hurt and my bike sucked. He was quiet for a minute, and I thought I was in for it for shouting and complaining, but all he did was point to his and Mom's bedroom, where it was dark, and our sole window air conditioning unit was running on high.

"Go lay down, I'll get you a drink of water."

I obeyed, too tired to argue or pretend I was fine. I laid back on the pillow and closed my eyes, feeling the vein in my forehead pulsing. Dad brought in water and a cool washcloth, which he laid over my eyes. I pulled the money out of my pocket, threw it on the mattress beside me, and fell immediately into a deep sleep.

Several hours later I awoke, as Dad came in and called my name.

"Magoo, you're supposed to be good at math, but I think you counted wrong. That pay wasn't so bad. More than I make."

He winked at me and told me there was supper if I wanted it, then he turned and left.

I rubbed my eyes, rolled over, and examined the bills I

had angrily tossed on the bed before passing out. I did a quick check and found twenty more dollars there than I thought I first calculated. Had I been wrong? Sweet relief filled me at the time, that I hadn't worked all week for so little.

Sweet realization fills me today, knowing my dad slipped his daughter half his allowance that afternoon. No, I did not have a father like those in the families I babysat for, but he was doing what he could with what he had.

CHAPTER 30
No More Sister and the Shift

Ever since I can remember, my eyes came to her shoulders, which had blades that sprung out on each side of her bony body like a bird's wings. If I stationed myself behind her, just inside those pinions, I could shelter from the scary music. You know, the "dun-dun-dun" before the door creaks open, the villain looks up and spots you, your eyes connect, and you know you're screwed.

My older sister is a complicated element of my past. She mothered me and bossed me, but mostly she served as my shield, as she did not have the self-preservation senses that I possessed. She either could not detect danger, or sometimes I think she chased it.

When we were younger, she simply didn't notice the potential for disaster, but in her teenage years, I believe she relished the debate. Either inadvertent or intentional, both led to doors slamming, tears shed, voices raised, and mayhem that could have been completely avoided with a few well-placed moves and buttoned-up lips.

In a thriller film, you watch in suspense, through the cracks in the fingers pressed over your eyes. You silently recite "Don't do it, don't open that door," under your breath like a mantra, but the main characters do, they always open the door. And she did, every time. She threw open the door, despite my attempts to whisper-shout her down or jab her in the ribs.

The positive outcome is that it took the focus off me. Many a day I slid into the background while those two clashed, one part of me relieved, and the other part all nervous stomach. For years I watched my sister fight the battle. She ran up against him so many times, the arguing, crying, and wreckage. I had learned that usually the best way was the soft way, skirt the trouble, and stay out of dodge. I became an expert at flying under the radar, which wasn't hard to do when the two of them were always at it.

But as my sister entered her later years of high school, she began to spend less and less time at home. At the height of their arguments, she would yell, "I'm outta here!"

Dad would reply, "Don't come back!"

And one day she didn't.

I waited all night to hear her car pull in, finally dozed off, and woke in the morning to see her twin bed in our shared room still made. I busied myself getting ready for school, keeping noise to a minimum as usual. Both Mom and Dad were sleeping, and it was best to keep it that way, in fact I had taken to swallowing a tablespoon of instant coffee with a glass of water instead of risking the sound of the microwave door waking anyone. I caught a ride to school with friends and tried not to think about the absence of my sister.

She showed up later that afternoon when I got home from school and told me she had stayed at a friend's house. It became a pattern, and more nights than not, she wasn't home. I learned later that she spent many nights sleeping in her car if a friend's couch wasn't an option, and by the time she graduated high school, she was regularly elsewhere.

At first it was peaceful without her there, pushing buttons and not backing down, but eventually and inevitably, the target rolled around to me. How would I survive without those bird blades to crouch behind and her irrational disregard for disaster? Would the spotlight now shine on me, a torch poking its beam into every crevice of my inadequacies?

When I entered adolescence there was a subtle yet certain shift. I began wearing girly clothes and doing my hair, and the first time Dad came into my bedroom and found me styling it with the curling iron, he let me know his displeasure.

"Oh Christ, not you too. Here, I thought I had one kid with some commonsense God gave 'em, but you're gonna turn out just like her."

He shook his head dramatically and left the room, and somehow his disappointment was worse than his anger.

I lived in constant paranoia that he would burst into my bedroom while I was changing, since there was no lock on the door. Our one bathroom offered even less privacy, as Dad demanded that the door stay cracked an inch, even when I was bathing. He said it was because steam would build up on the walls and ceiling.

Unlike my sister, I refused to argue about the excessive rules or any other topic, but instead, I would ignore him. This drove him crazy, because he wanted someone to debate with, and I wouldn't play the role. Oh, don't get me wrong, there were a few times that the F-bomb dropped out of my mouth, and it felt good, powerful, even during a heated exchange, but later I would feel tarnished. My usual response to trouble was to retreat inside myself or slip out the door.

Mentally, I began to separate everything about him that would not be the future me. The qualities in me that he doted on and praised, how I was his little sidekick who went on hikes, counted deer in fields, and appreciated nature, were discarded as if they had never been me. I claimed that looking at wildlife was for losers. I told myself to quit caring about all that stuff, but a love of the outdoors was instilled deep inside of me, and I knew that it would take more than a vow to expel it.

I also planned to be smarter than him. If the only way out of here was up and out, I would study as hard as I could and escape this place for university. If I became better educated, more successful, and moved miles away, could I outrun this life and the trappings of a controlling father and a disease no one would name?

I think he detected it. He sensed my uppity ways and how I thought I was too good for him now, so instead of sparring, we passed with a wide berth around each other in our small, shared space.

CHAPTER 31
Barnacle

Not since I competed in the New Glarus, Wisconsin regional spelling bee in the fifth grade, had my father attended another one of my events, which makes me think that this is when his physical symptoms must have become too difficult to hide in public. With Mom working the PM shift, no one came to school Christmas programs, academic award nights, or tennis tournaments, and she was a single parent at my high school graduation ceremony.

My friends' families always offered the extra seat in their vans, and I became the plus one everywhere I went. A guest at each house, I gratefully took the extra chair pulled out at every table, an additional place setting who was never any trouble. I spooned up the vegetables that my friends complained about eating, and I always used my manners and offered to help clean up after. My friends would roll their eyes and say, "Gee thanks, you're making us look bad!", but their parents loved me, and I soaked up the affection.

One special family frequently stowed me in the back seat of their Ford sedan for long summer weekends, and it was only a matter of time before their daughter invited me to come to summer camp with her.

"You can ride with me and my family," she said. "It'll be fun. Plus, there's always cute boys at camp." She smiled convincingly.

Well, she had me at cute boys, but then I swallowed and had to ask, "How much does it cost?"

She handed me a flyer, and when I looked at the rate for a week at sleep-away-camp, I gulped. That was more money than I had saved at any one time, and I knew there was no way my family was going to be able, or willing, to pay for it.

"I'll think about it," I said.

"Please, please come," she begged.

"I'll try," I said.

I ramped up the babysitting and tucked away every spare dollar I could earn. Soon it was close to the deadline for signing up, and I had almost saved enough but wasn't completely there. I filled out the registration form anyway and with suspended breath, brought it to Mom and asked if I could go.

She held the brochure, giving it a once-over, and when her eyes reached the cost, she looked up at me in alarm.

"I have almost all of it saved," I said.

She looked relieved but still narrowed her eyes.

"How much have you got?"

I told her how close I was, and she said she thought she could manage the rest, so I sent in the paperwork. I couldn't believe it was really going to happen, one whole week away from home.

CHAPTER 32
Camp

Sleep-away camp in the central woods of Wisconsin was filled with the smells of sand and pine and the anticipation of adventure. As we pulled into the gravel turn-around and began unloading our gear, I filled with apprehension and anxiety. What if these kids aren't friendly? What if they can tell I'm different?

I had nothing to fear. Before we finished unpacking our things, campers from years past surrounded the vehicle, all wanting to catch up with my friend. Her grandfather was a pastor and had helped found this camp, so she and her family were well known by staff and campers alike. She'd been coming here since she was a little kid, and it seemed like she knew everyone.

She quickly introduced me, and the rest was easy. Turns out, I could throw on a bucket hat and a denim jacket and be warmly accepted into this circle. It didn't matter that my dad didn't work a real job and was angry, fidgety, and weird, that no one was allowed to come over to my house, and that my clothes were hand-me-downs from Mom's boss's daughter. At camp I had a fresh start, and the relief made me feel light, like I had set something heavy down, and I kept fighting the urge to check if I had dropped something I was supposed to be carrying.

My cabin counselor was a college student from South Dakota, and I was enamored with her coolness. She seemed to truly get me, and she said she wanted to understand my problems, so one night before lights out, we sat on our bunks, and I cracked open. I told her about my dad and how angry and strange he behaved, how everyone thought he was crazy, but no one talked about it or did anything about it. I admittedly downplayed the possibility of genetic illness, because saying it aloud made it real. Likely what came out of my mouth was typical pre-teen angst, to which she gave the advice of listening to Pop Christian music loudly on your headphones and praying for peace. I don't blame her. I might have given similar guidance in her shoes.

Camp was filled with water sports, craft time, meals in the dining hall, and campfire singalongs. An American Baptist camp, it was also filled with daily Bible study, vespers worship services, and lots of Jesus everywhere.

I left camp that week transformed. At the final campfire, there was an altar call. I walked up and committed my life to Jesus in a way that had never happened before, certainly not in the dank basement of the church Mom took us to. As much as my adolescent mind could understand, I believed God would hear me when I called, and I planned to hold Him to that promise once I got back home.

There were tears and more tears and plenty of hugging when the week ended. We campers had formed friendships stronger than steel and pledged to write letters and stay in touch until next year. As the car wound its way back to my hometown, I couldn't help but wonder if things would be different. I certainly felt changed, but was it simply because I'd had a week where I could breathe?

My friend's family dropped me off at my driveway, and I declined the offer from her dad to help me carry my things up the green steps.

"No thank you, I've got it. Thank you so much again!" I waved as they drove off.

I trudged up the steps, making several trips until my sleeping bag and luggage were settled on "The Green." Then, and only then, did I try the door. It was locked.

I knocked hesitantly, knowing this would set him off. No answer.

I rapped louder, calling out, "It's me, I'm here!"

Finally, after what seemed forever, I heard shuffling in the kitchen, the curtain moving to the side as the peephole was checked. Dad unlocked the door and swung it open.

"Well, look what dragged in," he said by way of greeting, looking like he had just woken up, his hair all over the place, but at least wearing briefs.

I cast my eyes away from him and started carrying my things in. Everything looked messier, darker, and dustier than before I left if that was even possible.

"Hi Dad, I'm home," I tried for the cheery approach.

"I can see that," he said with little to no emotion. He took in my tanned skin and arms filled with hand-tied friendship bracelets.

"How was church camp?" he asked, but the tone of his voice showed he didn't mean it sincerely. Five minutes in the door, and he was already priming for a fight.

I didn't take the bait. "It was good. You know, I think things are going to be different around here. I'm different," I announced.

"Oh yeah, well you don't look very different to me," he said.

Against my better judgement I told him. I said that I was a Christian and was going to live a life of love to others. He would see a difference in me, and I hoped we'd get along better from now on.

Before I had even finished, he was bent over, cackling. After he wiped his eyes, he switched and looked at me with intensity.

"We'll just see about that, won't we? We'll see if you are any better."

CHAPTER 33
The Tennis Bus

"Okay, good match tonight. See you at practice tomorrow afternoon," Coach said.

The bus slid briefly off to the side of the road, and the doors opened. I slipped out like a shadow, and took off down the sidewalk, tennis bag slung over my shoulder. I didn't look back, but I knew the bus would shove off quickly, as if it had never stopped. It was a bit of a favor, my coach looking the other way and pausing the bus enroute to the high school, where he parked it after weeknight away matches.

Parents waited in the parking lot in their station wagons, and upper-class students had left their cars or scooters there. It was likely against school rules, the athletic code, and all sorts of common sense to drop kids off at their houses, but Coach knew that I would walk home in the dark otherwise, and he didn't want that. The first time he offered to drop me, the panic must have shone in my eyes.

My sophomore year in high school was my first year on the tennis team, and the first thing I had ever been allowed to do. After my sister moved out, my parents started to relax. Often my father didn't even notice whether I was around, as long as I kept a low profile. Being ignored was sweet relief, and being on this team was the closest thing to normal I had ever been a part of. I didn't want to mess it up for anything.

When Coach suggested, I said "Maybe just at the corner, then you, you wouldn't have to go out of your way or anything?" My eyes pleaded with him to understand and not ask questions.

He casually nodded in agreement, "Yeah, that could work."

Did he know? Could he imagine the hole I would want to crawl into if that bus full of athletes pulled up to my house? If everyone, including the superior seniors, witnessed what I called home or saw my dad sitting on the porch in his underwear? Whether Coach had guessed any of that or not, a plan was made to drop me at the corner, and I think we both breathed a collective sigh of relief to have successfully skirted that awkward topic.

This night was like most others at 10:00 PM in my neighborhood, a block of run-down duplexes and small homes which hovered next to the central railroad changing yard of our city. Over the years my sleep had become accustomed to the sounds of the train cars colliding as the night shift engineers connected one line to another, re-routing the tracks, and sending rail cars south to Chicago or east to Milwaukee.

Sometimes, a train raced through with more cars than I could count, logs strapped on their backs and bound for the northern paper companies. When we were younger, my sister and I would sit on the sidewalk and feel our bottoms vibrate as those cars flew through. I used to imagine that, if I could somehow grab hold, I could ride those logs like a wild horse, escape this town and head north for adventure.

I hiked my tennis bag up on my shoulder and shook my head, remembering the silly dreams of running away which were borderline obsessions during most of my childhood. I knew now that the only tangible way to fly away was to study hard and bide your time. Keep your mouth shut and don't make trouble. But it grated on me still, it felt like giving in, and playing the game. Riding that lumber would have made for a much more dramatic exit.

CHAPTER 34
Neighborhood Admirer

I had a secret admirer. Every summer I rode my bike each week over to Grandpa and Grandma's house to mow their lawn and do other jobs, like gardening or cleaning, for some extra cash to finance the never ending "keeping up with my friends fund." Little did I know that when I mowed the vacant lot next door to their home, a neighbor boy named Chris down the street was also cutting the grass and looking over to see the girl.

Chris and his family lived four houses down from Grandpa and Grandma, and his whole growing up he knew them and found them to be eccentric. He tells the story about riding his bike on the dirt trail that ran across Grandpa's property. My grandpa refused to pay the tax assessment to have pavement put in. He didn't agree with the price the City wanted to charge and therefore, it remained unfinished, and he would approach City Hall at any point in time, should anyone wish to discuss it, and argue his point until the end. I do believe the City gave up on him and decided that there were bigger fish to fry than Grandpa's sidewalk.

My grandfather was the mayor of our small town in 1950, for which he was elected to one term, and he then went on to serve as Assemblyman in the Independent Party for multiple terms thereafter. Even when Grandpa's political career ended, he continued to fight the good fight, always one to dissertate on public affairs whether you had asked or not.

Chris remembers trick or treating with the neighbor kids at my grandma's house and how it was always a complicated ordeal. You had to come into the kitchen and show her your costume, say where you lived, what your name was, and who your parents were. Then finally you'd get your candy and be on your way. He remembers my grandma always dressed like a witch, and that she would sway back and forth in her flowing costume and pointy hat, always smiling wide, almost scary wide.

When you live in a small town with one high school, everyone knows everyone, so I had heard of this boy, but we hadn't had any classes together. It wasn't too long before we crossed paths at the local grocery store just down the street from Grandpa and Grandma's house where Chris was a bagger, and I had recently landed a job running the cash register.

He kept his light brown hair longer in the back, and I would see him frequently pull a black pocket comb from his

Bugle Boy khakis to feather the sides. His eyes were an even deeper brown, paired with a mischievous grin and the signature red bowtie of the store's uniform. As I would shoot the goods down the conveyor belt, he scooped them into paper sacks, and we got to know each other. We joked around, found we had some chemistry, and Chris worked up the courage to ask me out. With a little bit of negotiation and charm, I agreed to a first date, and after that we became inseparable.

Chris's family took me in. Most days after school, he and I would finish our homework at his house, then head over to the grocery store for our shift, come back for a frozen pizza and a TV show, and then he would drive me home.

I spent as little time at my house as possible during the rest of my high school years. I slept there, grabbed a bite to eat or a cup of coffee, and headed out the door. Chris knew that my dad was difficult, but I kept my guard up and only told him the most basic facts. I really liked this guy and didn't want to wreck it.

In 1987 Great Aunt Eilene was the first sister to lose her battle with Huntington's Disease at 60 years of age. I remember little about the funeral, other than it being Catholic, with strange words and a canister of smoke, which the priest swung around on a chain. I remember hushed words among the family members, of how bad it had gotten while Eilene was away in

Colorado, how no one realized it had gotten that bad. There was talk that her son had it too, Dad's cousin and friend, who he used to run around our town with. Everyone whispered and called it "It."

I was terrified of HD, but also in the first stages of love, and those euphoric feelings overrode the fear and despair, so I gladly escaped to them instead. Chris and I spent every free minute together. When we were not at our sports practices and competitions, him track and cross country and me tennis, then we worked our jobs at the grocery store, studied, and went to school together.

This state of buffered bliss couldn't have lasted forever, eventually he would have to meet my parents. The night he planned to introduce himself to my dad, I was terrified.

"Well at least his name isn't Jason," Dad smiled, teasing me, and thoroughly enjoying himself while doing so.

"Dad! Do not even say that!"

I ran around the house, trying to tidy without him noticing that I was moving things, as rearranging anything was usually strictly forbidden in the "Book of Dad." I wished I could open the curtains and let in some light, but I knew that would be a hard no. Yes, I had the unfortunate record of dating not one, not two, but three Jason's in succession, and although my father only met one of them, he delighted in reminding me of it.

I saw through the home-made peephole that Chris was

climbing the outside steps, and my pulse quickened. He paused on "The Green," and I opened the door for him before he could knock.

"Nice to meet you sir," Chris held out his hand, and he and my dad shook, a firm grip. Thank God Dad was at least wearing more than underwear. He wore a faded but presentable T-shirt and a pair of sweatpants, and his hair, wet from the bath, was slicked back.

It turned out they had a lot in common. Dad and Chris started talking, first about hunting, then moved to fishing, and before long, it was country roads and Dad's favorite topic, Zander's Lake, and Cadiz Springs.

"Okay Dad, can I have my boyfriend now?" I finally interrupted them just as Dad was warming up to his junking route and his van, and I sensed a tour coming. Too much information.

We escaped outside and down the steps with Dad holding the door and shouting down to come back anytime.

"Your dad's not so bad," Chris said, looking over at me and smiling, one hand on the steering wheel and the other holding mine.

I smiled back at him. What did this mean? Dared I hope that my dad was just odd and shifty, that this wasn't Huntington's disease slowly invading? Could I have a normal future, a happy forever after with this guy? Or was Chris just being nice, trying to make me feel better?

He had only experienced the smallest taste, less than fifteen minutes of Dad in his almost best mood and tamed behavior. I wasn't sure, but perhaps increasing the dose slowly was my most feasible plan.

CHAPTER 35
Intersecting Circles

My remaining years of high school were filled with Chris, tennis, and returning to camp each summer. I took advanced classes and earned straight A's each semester. My senior year I was the yearbook editor and had an extensive list of extracurriculars on my scholarship applications. I hadn't changed my mind about getting up and out, but now I had conflicting desires.

Chris rekindled my love for the outdoors, and we spent our free time driving country roads, spotting deer, even hiking around the lake at Cadiz Springs. "The Green" had been my playroom as a child, a respite in times of family conflict, but now it was where Chris and I stretched out on our backs, talking about anything and everything, and seeking much needed privacy. I was scared to admit how much he had come to mean to me, and questioned if you could find "the one" at such a young age. My parents had married young, and I wasn't sure I wanted to repeat their struggle.

True to the plan, Chris slowly but surely worked his way into our home and my family's heart, learning lessons from the "Book of Dad," such as how late to bring home his daughter (not past midnight), who can change the TV channel (only him), and the proper way to crush and dispose of an empty RC Cola can (more steps than you would think.) Chris took it all in stride, but he had yet to be introduced to the villain HD, and I was convinced that this would be what would send us our separate ways.

As we continued to grow closer my mind raced with hypotheticals. What if I had Huntington's disease? How could I expect Chris to care for me if I became confined to a wheelchair or trapped in a nursing home bed? What if I started acting obsessed and angry like my dad and drove him away? I didn't want a marriage like my parents had, and I couldn't bear the rejection if Chris decided to opt out first.

I made up my mind that I was going to end our relationship before he could, planning it for when I left for college out of state. After graduating, I would travel as far away from Wisconsin as scholarships would carry me, landing in Sioux Falls, South Dakota, where my camp counselors had all attended. This small private college was the Promised Land for a kid like me, who found love and acceptance at camp each summer from seventh grade until my Senior year. Those student counselors with bright faces assured me that this would be a place where I could shine.

Chris and I agreed to simply enjoy the summer of our senior year and see where life would take us after that. I convinced him that he should apply to college as well, and he was accepted at UW-Stevens Point. We both took summer jobs away from the grocery store to earn more tuition money, he worked at a cheese factory, and I was hired as a nursing assistant at a local long-term care facility.

Coincidentally, Chris's mother worked at this same nursing home, and it was also where Great Aunt Luanne received care, and for several years my Great Uncle Teddy lived there too.

When my great grandfather, who was their only living parent, passed away, Luanne and Teddy stayed at the family home. My cousin Bea recalls that Luanne took care of Teddy as long as she could, but in her late twenties, Great Aunt Luanne began showing physical signs of HD, which progressed quickly. Her siblings needed to find an option for both adult children with unique needs.

Bea remembers being at the farm as a child and hearing Luanne coming down the lane, her foot stomping and releasing the gas pedal with her involuntary movements, and my mother remembers watching Luanne careen around the town square. When Luanne eventually lost her driver's license, she and Teddy went to live at the nursing home. Later Teddy was placed in a group home for adults with developmental disabilities, but Luanne would remain a lifelong resident of this long-term care facility.

When Chris came with me to the farm that year for Easter, my relatives were in for a surprise. Chris spotted Teddy across the room, and their eyes connected in recognition.

"Hey Teddy, what's up? Wanna arm-wrestle?"

Chris slapped Great Uncle Teddy on the shoulder and sat down next to him at his card table for one. The family watched in shocked amazement as my boyfriend grabbed hold of Teddy's hand, and they went at it, Chris grunting and struggling, and then feigning defeat, much to Teddy's delight.

Then Chris had some explaining to do. He told them how he had spent countless hours at the nursing home, attended Christmas parties, brought his mom her supper, and picked her up after her shift when he had borrowed the car. He had been arm-wrestling Teddy for years, listening to him play his harmonica, and it seemed he'd known him almost as long as I had. This was more than a small-town coincidence. I asked myself, "Who was this guy, and how had he come into my life?"

To say that Chris was accepted into the extended family after that encounter was an understatement, and I both loved it and dreaded what was next, because if he knew Teddy, then surely everyone would soon be putting two and two together, and the scariest secret in my family would be exposed. Luanne.

Between our jobs and hanging out with friends, that summer after graduation flew by, and I could physically sense the clock ticking down. Against all rules in the "Book of Dad," my father didn't say a word when the night before I was to leave for university, Chris stayed way into the wee hours, and we kept my bedroom door closed.

Chris didn't understand why we needed to end our relationship. Over the summer we'd had small, careful conversations about Huntington's disease, and he claimed there was no way I had it. Even if I did, it would be years before anything would happen. Look at my grandma, he reasoned. She seemed fine, and we knew enough medical facts to know that she had to have it for my dad to, and then for me to. Despite my father's bizarre behavior, there was no proof that he had HD. Chris repeated all my assurances back to me.

"But we'll be so far away from each other," I said.

"Who cares if we're 1,000 miles apart! We'll write letters and call on the phone." His eyes were wet.

"I need to get away from here, far away from all of this," I said.

Now we both cried, said we loved each other, and I ended it.

CHAPTER 36
Cross Country in the RV

The following morning my grandpa and grandma drove me to South Dakota with all my stuff crammed in their travel trailer, and I imagined we would look like the Clampett's pulling into the campus parking lot. I moped every mile of that journey, gazing out the window and wondering, "What had I done?"

I had cut my only lifeline, the one person who truly understood me and my family. In those summer months before we went our separate ways, Chris and I spent more time at my house than ever before, even easing into a routine of dinner there, a couple of nights a week.

Dad had eased up about us being in the kitchen, and things had been going smoothly until one August weekend before I left, he exploded over something Mom did or said. I cannot even remember what triggered him, but it was an all-out brawl. As their shouting increased in volume, Chris observed me shrinking in demeanor and suggested we sit on the porch and wait it out.

How many times as a child had I sat on this green carpet, plugging my ears, and floating away? Although tonight I had a hand to hold, the shame and embarrassment was crippling. Chris's family wasn't perfect, but they had never exchanged harsh words in front of me, not once.

Chris tried to comfort me, promising it would blow over soon, but once he saw me visibly shaking, he knew he needed to get me out of there. We went back into the kitchen to get our jackets in time to witness Dad put his fist through their bedroom door. His eyes were wild and unfocused, and a sweaty film coated his forehead. Mom was nowhere to be seen, probably hiding in my bedroom. Chris grabbed our coats, and we exited quickly and quietly.

"Is that what it's like when it's bad?" Chris asked once we were in his car and driving aimlessly around our town.

"Yes, and so much worse," I said, not meeting his gaze.

I didn't have anywhere to hide, no excuses to make, and I was tired of coming up with them. It felt freeing, like a weight was being lifted, that finally someone knew what happened in my home. I proceeded to tell him about the angry outbursts that were more common than not, how minor changes in routine mysteriously triggered Dad's fury. I admitted that I had to lobby with him to put on clothes if Chris was coming over, otherwise most days he was walking around in nothing while I awkwardly tried to avert my eyes.

Recently Dad threatened suicide, said he was going to drive the car into a brick wall, with my mom in it. He was up every night, pacing, talking in pressured speech to himself or anyone who would listen. He kept the TV on at all hours, and it was impossible to get any sleep. During the day our apartment remained dark, dusty curtains closed, Mom and I tiptoeing around so as not to wake the giant. The three of us were more isolated than ever, no one was allowed in, nor would I want anyone to be. I was suffocating slowly.

Chris's jaw set tight, and he pulled over.

"You don't need to be ashamed. None of this is your fault," Chris said and held me while I cried.

The hole in my parent's bedroom door was a constant reminder, for the remainder of the summer, that my family was broken, and I told myself that I didn't deserve a guy like Chris. If it was HD that made my dad act this way, would he get worse? If I got HD, would I then act like him? My sister was already gone, and I would soon escape as well, but what about my mom? I wondered and worried how she was going to survive in that house alone when I left for college.

After over nine hours cross country, Grandpa pulled his big rig up to my new home. I saw students strolling the grounds, some groups sitting on blankets under aged oak trees, others tossing a football back and forth. I saw large brick buildings steeped in academia, and I could barely contain my excitement. Yes, I already missed Chris so much that it physically hurt, but this was my fresh start. Could I have both?

Mom had come along for the trip, and we carried box after box to my floor and unpacked. Once I was settled into my dorm, she looked around wistfully, as if she wished she could also enroll as opposed to returning east to her life with Dad. She hugged me and handed me an MCI long distance calling card.

"Make it last," she said, "and keep in touch."

"I will," I promised.

That night I punched the long code from the back of the card into the shared telephone which hung in our student lobby. I stretched the cord around the corner for privacy and waited. After a series of beeps, it rang and finally connected, and I heard his voice say hello.

"I don't want to break up!" I choked out in one exhaled breath before he could say anything else.

There it was, hanging in all its vulnerability. He could have said he'd already moved on, that I had been right, and we shouldn't risk a relationship with how crazy my dad was or the threat of HD in my future. He paused, and the silence, but for the crackling on the line, felt eternal.

"Okay, that's the best news ever," he said, and I could hear the relief in his voice.

We then crammed as many words as we could into the next ten minutes, conserving the calling card, and ended with "I love you's", a long-distance relationship, and a 116-day countdown until Christmas break.

CHAPTER 37
Preliminary Research

I entered the campus library nervously, and moved to the back of the stacks where the research section was. There were shelves upon shelves of leatherbound anthologies and tables holding Microfiche machines, which I have always hated. The idea of pressing your forehead up against the same panel that every other greasy forehead had pressed up against, and scanning through the black and white discs while zooming in and out made me motion sick. I hoped the information I was looking for wasn't stored on Microfiche. Truth be told I hoped the information I was looking for wasn't in this library.

A young librarian student-worker approached and asked if she could help me find something. I reluctantly inquired on a section for hereditary diseases and neurological illnesses.

"Are you a bio major?" the perky librarian asked. "I haven't seen you in here before."

"Are you writing a book, or do you just shelve them?" I thought to myself. She looked at me inquisitively, and her eyes narrowed. Shoot, had I said that aloud? But no, I hadn't, and her eyes brightened back up.

"Never mind, let's get you settled," she said.

I pulled a heavy volume, its contents in mouse font. Since I was pretty sure "The Shakes" wasn't in the index, I looked under H for Huntington's, and there it was, "Huntington's disease."

I couldn't breathe.

For the next three hours I pored over the material, medical facts with large numbers and words I had to look up in the dictionary. Much of what I read confirmed what Grandma had been telling me over the years. I could picture her notes, but somehow seeing it outside of her clumsy jangled script made it more real.

The genetic information I gleaned from those textbooks in 1990 was limited, as the HD gene wasn't discovered until 1993. Predictive testing for Huntington's disease became available in 1986 using linkage analysis, finding genetic markers of the condition within a family. Scientific mapping based on clinical observations and hereditary research had determined its autosomal dominance, meaning that individuals with an affected parent had a 50% chance of inheriting the mutated gene. In simple terms, if Dad had HD, I was a coin flip.

I read about chorea, involuntary movements which were a result of the degeneration of the basal ganglia, the part of the brain that governs motor control. I learned there was no cure, no test, and I compiled a laundry list of psychological symptoms which described my father to a tee. Almost all people with HD will manifest personality and behavioral changes as part of what might be called hypo frontal or dysexecutive syndrome, characterized by apathy, irritability, impulsivity, and obsessionality.

Uncontrolled movements, obsessive behavior, angry outbursts, depression, insomnia, and oh my God, the inability to regulate their own body temperature, causing those affected to shed clothing, sometimes inappropriately. I don't know if I felt better or worse that there was a scientific reason for my dad's constant and embarrassing nakedness.

From a cross-reference I then slipped into the rabbit hole of Woody Guthrie, the most famous person associated with Huntington's disease. Guthrie, a legendary folk singer, known for his ballads and poetry, died from HD complications just three years before I was born. I read about his bouts of rage and paranoia, which hit too close to home, and his commitment to a mental institution in 1956, which terrified me.

Guthrie's wife Marjorie worked tirelessly after his death to raise awareness and founded the Huntington's Disease Society of America (HDSA.) This was the association that my grandmother was always talking about. I closed my eyes and remembered plucking the chords to "This Land is Your Land" as a young girl. Grandma had bought both my sister and me acoustic guitars for Christmas one year, and she smiled and tapped her toe when I learned and then played that song for her. Had she known that the author and composer was affected with HD? Is that why her smile had seemed wistful at the time?

Perhaps the most difficult fact I found in all of the resource materials was inconsistency. At the time of this research, the age of Huntington's onset varied significantly, even among members of the same family. The severity of the symptoms affected each person differently, and the pace of decline could not be predicted. This wasn't what I wanted to hear. This meant that my grandmother could have mild, slowly progressing HD, my dad could have a raging case with psychological symptoms that had started early in his life, and I could be at-risk for anything in between. I closed the books, returned to my dorm room, and curled up under the covers.

86 days until Christmas break.

CHAPTER 38
A Pebble and a Peninsula

My freshman year at this conservative faith-based university was a bit like being a foreign exchange student in another country. These shiny, happy people had no idea the boulder I was carrying, but it wasn't their fault. I hadn't shared with anyone here about what was happening at home, because there was something about them that I didn't understand or trust. Their language was filled with hope and happiness, and believing the future is in God's control.

I wondered, "If God was in control of this train wreck of my life, what kind of God was that?" but I couldn't come out and say it. My arm was once again as heavy as lead in a Sunday school classroom, devoid of acceptable answers and unable to express my doubts and frustrations at their eternal optimism.

I did find a few close friends and then began to flourish in Creative Writing 101. The prompts were interesting, I had no one to impress, and nothing to lose, so I wrote authentically and honestly. After the first assignment was handed back, my professor and I built a rapport. He always told me he couldn't wait to see what I would write next, and teased me about never turning in rough drafts, even if that was the assignment. He encouraged me to write for the school paper, and I said I'd think about it.

Every Wednesday morning at 8:00 AM was Chapel, listed as optional in the university announcements, but everyone went to Chapel, and those students who skipped were looked down upon. So, when I'd rather be sleeping in with the duvet pulled over my head, I would drag out, drink a coffee, and head over to the ministry building. That morning the topic was relationships, and our campus pastor went retro, channeling Simon and Garfunkel to make the case that no one is a rock, and no one is an island. I appreciated everything he had to say. He wasn't wrong.

And yet later that day an idea built in my head for an article for the paper. Whether it was late at night, or I was feeling more cynical than usual, I produced a satirical piece that evening called "A Pebble and a Peninsula," the premise being that yes, Pastor was right. We can't be rocks. We can't be islands. But do we have to be so happy at 7:00 AM in the community bathroom? Do I have to smile at everyone brushing their teeth? Couldn't we have a little bit of space around here? Couldn't I be a pebble or a peninsula?

Oh boy, did I rock waves like a high surf on the West Coast. The girls on my floor were hurt and offended, and it created so much silent treatment and drama, I can't recount it without cringing. I apologized to several classmates on my floor and to the pastor who delivered the original message. He said he understood and found my piece witty and humorous, sort of.

This university wasn't summer camp, and I had fled here for all the wrong reasons. Between the flop of the article and my heart caving and crashing with missing Chris, it was clear that I wasn't going to be able to stay here much longer. Problem being, I didn't want to go home.

15 days until Christmas break.

I carpooled back to Wisconsin for Christmas with some other students in a van with no heat. I couldn't feel my feet by the time we arrived at the park and ride where Chris was waiting, engine running. I was overwhelmed with joy as I saw him standing there in his letter jacket, smiling at me, but I was also a little nervous. How would it be to see him in person again? I hadn't shared any of my research or fears in our letters and phone calls.

I thanked the friends, and Chris grabbed my bags and

stowed them in the back, while I climbed in and scooted all the way over to his side, kicking off my penny loafers, and cranking up the heat.

He drove with one arm on the wheel and the other around my shoulders. We immediately picked up where we had left off, and even though we were headed back to our hometown and whatever nightmare might be waiting, I felt safe in his arms. I planned to pick up some shifts at the nursing home, but other than that, we had twenty whole days to spend together.

CHAPTER 39
Seniority

"Okay, Luanne, let's get you clean."

I picked her up like a small child, and she whimpered softly, inhaling, and exhaling noisily through her nose as I transferred her thin, naked body from the bed to the shower chair. The sour smell of urine hit my nostrils, and her underarm sweat soaked into my uniform.

We were short staffed, it was late, and I had a dozen more residents to put to bed after this shower. At least it was Luanne. I could have been assigned Phil, who snickered when you scrubbed between his legs and tried to grab your bottom if you became distracted while adjusting the sprayer.

Luanne wouldn't complain that I hadn't reached all the important parts. She wouldn't argue or talk back. The biggest challenge with Luanne was making sure she didn't shimmy out of this shower chair on wheels.

I wrapped her up tightly in a bath sheet, and we exited her room and headed down the hall towards the shower room. No matter how tightly I swaddled her, Luanne's arms would somehow Houdini out of the towel and begin flailing around, and she involuntarily backhanded me across the face as I attempted to re-adjust the bath sheet. The cloth slipped off revealing bare shoulders, a puddle of liquid grew on the floor as she wet herself through the hole in the shower chair, and I became desperate.

Giving up all pretense of modesty, we made a break for our destination, navigating through the narrow entrance of the shower room as, not only her arms, but now her legs had broken free of the towel and waved wildly.

This long-term care facility where I picked up hours during summer breaks and holiday vacations was constantly struggling. The universal reason for every cut corner and low standard was the budget. I often wondered what actually was in the budget, because any need or issue that was brought to administration was simply deemed not in it.

Better shower facilities were not in the budget, and it took forever to get the water temperature regulated with this relic of a faucet. Tonight, the handle was proving more difficult than usual, and Luanne was agitated and shivering by the time I coaxed the water warm enough for her to get in. Once wet she became even more slippery, and although I would have been thrilled for an extra pair of hands to hold her in place, those weren't in the budget either.

My grandmother had told me how reassured she felt, knowing I was home for the holiday. Last week when I stopped by, she patted my cheek, and said, "Bless you, child, Luanne is in good hands."

For Grandma, I robbed a few extra minutes from the next resident on my list and took my time, shampooing her sister's once-black hair, now salted with gray, and speckled with dandruff, clipped in a no-nonsense haircut, and standing on end.

As my fingers massaged her scalp, I imagined what she must have looked like as a young girl, my age. I wondered if she wore fire-engine red lipstick like my grandmother or painted her nails like Great Aunt Harriet. Did she style her hair with hot rollers and tie a scarf at her neck?

I thought about the picture collage I used to gaze at, the five sisters at the farm, and it was hard to believe that Luanne had ever held still long enough to pose for a photo. My dad had bestowed her with her nickname, and the entire extended family still affectionately referred to Luanne as "String Bean."

"Skin and bones that one was," my father said of the great aunt I would never really know, "and the name just stuck."

I pictured her working at the telephone company, fingers flying as she connected each caller to their destination socket. I bet she never figured her fingers would fly as they do now, out of control and non-stop, burning calories each waking hour. My grandmother remembers Luanne was beautiful and told me she had been dating a handsome beau before her symptoms started.

It was inconceivable that in her late twenties, "Bean" began to shake and move, her body withered, and she eventually entered this nursing home, never to leave.

Luanne had seniority in this facility. She would spend over thirty years of her life here, her brain cells slowly deteriorating. She lost control of her arms and legs, her ability to communicate and feed herself, to use the bathroom independently, and maintain her dignity.

This is what Huntington's disease looks like, I pondered, at worst-case scenario. This terminal genetic illness kills you as slowly as a glacier, those massive sheets of ice which, scouring the surface of our earth, forever alter its landscape. Risk was in my face, at first terrifying, then hypnotically washing over me.

I startled from my reverie when I heard it, a scream strangled and mutated, one only a non-verbal person can make. She was scalding. Frantically, I turned the temperature gauge, first one way, then the other to no avail, as she thrashed in the shower chair, her cries echoing off the bathroom walls. Giving up on the worthless knob, I wrenched her shower chair out of the steaming spray and wrapped her in a towel. Soap remained in her hair.

I couldn't speak. I was shaking, and my heart pounded in

my chest as if it might force itself out onto the shower floor at any minute. I held all ninety pounds of my great aunt in my arms and felt her wetness soak into my scrubs for the second time that night. I checked her over for superficial burns, but thankfully she was unharmed. Eventually her sobs subsided, although she continued to struggle against me, and I wasn't sure if it was intentional or not.

"I'm sorry. I'm so sorry," I whispered to Luanne.

"Grandma, I'm sorry I let you down," I thought to myself as well.

"What was that all about?" the floor nurse called from across the hall, looking up from her charts as we exited the shower and wheeled back to Luanne's room.

"Nothing," I said.

I shrugged off her raised eyebrows and kept going. I focused on getting Luanne in bed with blinders on, ignoring the jokes and banter of the other nurse's aides as they tackled the PM shift, popping worn and wrinkled bodies into their beds like coins into slots.

I positioned the plastic mattress pad under Luanne, tied the gown loosely around the back of her neck, and attempted to smooth her damp hair and wipe away the leftover suds. As I lifted the bed rail, she settled into small twitches and soon would drift off, then succumb to deep sleep, the only time her limbs fell completely still.

I remained by the bed, longing to rewind this evening, to edit just a few small but significant parts. Better yet, I ached to edit history, and swap just a few small strands of genetic code.

179

CHAPTER 40
Someone Else's Story

My shifts caring for Luanne were a reality check, and before leaving for the Spring term I shared everything I had learned to date about Huntington's with Chris, as well as my fears that my dad had it, and I would get it too. He continued to assure me that he loved me, and no disease would change that.

After yet another tearful goodbye, Chris and I started a fresh countdown until I would visit him at his school over Spring Break. I boarded a Greyhound bus back west, both resolved and conflicted. Some days I was committed to making every moment count, other days convinced that I had symptoms already, so what was the point? I was easily spooked by tripping or clumsiness, and I obsessed and worried about every mishap. On campus, I was constantly paranoid that others would notice any abnormal behavior. What originally attracted me to this out-of-state school was an opportunity to reinvent myself and shed HD and my family like a snakeskin.

Then I got a wild idea to tell all.

I stood in front of Freshman Public Speaking 101, holding the two three-by-five index cards permitted and too late to turn back now. It was Monday, 8:30 AM, and my fellow students passed time by sleeping, whispering with one another, or last-minute crafting of their own speeches. The assignment was to use a shocking introductory statement to grab the audience's attention.

"Over holiday break I watched my Great Aunt Luanne die," I said.

Okay, I had their attention.

For the next three and a half minutes, I lifted the veil for these strangers. I relived the months post-graduation and most recently on holiday break, working as a nursing assistant for the long-term care facility in my hometown. I told them about Huntington's disease and what it does, slowly and methodically, to your mind and body. I shared my research and then the underbelly, my own risk.

Because I did not really know these people, I tossed out all the dark possibilities. I had spent my shifts caring for Luanne, who was end-stage and my grandmother's sister. If Grandma also carried the gene, she could pass it to my dad. If Dad had HD, there was a 50% chance I did too, the gift that keeps giving. There, I said it aloud, for the first time.

Crickets.

After my conclusion, you could have heard a pin drop. A couple people cleared their throats, most looked down, around, anywhere else. I do not know that I finished as strong as I started. By nature, my story kind of tapers off, and you are left asking, "Now what?"

"Alright, everyone, we're done for today," the professor said.

He rattled off last minute instructions for next week in his nasal monotone, and everyone jumped at the chance to flee. Binders slammed shut, backpacks zipped, and conversations resumed right where they left off. Who was going out later, and what chances did the basketball team have against our rival this weekend. The room cleared, and not a trace of Luanne remained. Like unmarked graves these empty desks blinked back at me.

I realized that, for all the upturned faces and concerned looks, in the end, my speech was just someone else's story. Like the infomercials on television displaying African orphans with protruding bellies and sad brown eyes. You feel convicted for a moment, you ponder what you can do, and then you change the channel, because it is making you uncomfortable.

23 days until Spring Break.

CHAPTER 41
First Proposal

We laid in his upper loft, and I was fighting the claustrophobia of being inches from the ceiling of Chris's dorm room. We studied the stucco and held hands. I had to leave today, catching a ride with friends back to South Dakota. We cautiously talked of the future, skirting the topic of illness and risk.

Suddenly, Chris shot up, so quickly that I thought he might hit his head on the ceiling. He took both of my hands in his.

"I don't have a ring, I don't know what the future holds, but I do know one thing – I love you, and I want to spend the rest of our lives together, however long we get."

His brown eyes laser focused on mine.

"If I asked you to marry me, would you say yes?" He asked.

So serious. Dead serious, I thought, then stopped. Too much thinking was often a problem for me. This man knew everything, as much everything as I had been willing to share and even more that had leaked out despite my best efforts to keep it in. His love was unconditional.

"Yes. If you asked me, I would say yes," I answered him, and he held me close.

What had I done? Was it fair of me to say yes to him? To commit to spending our lives together when we knew how badly it could go? I felt elated and selfish at the same time, no two more unrelated emotions had co-existed in my heart. And what would everyone else think? Would they judge me as self-seeking, entrapping this good man to a future of the "in sickness" part of the marriage vows?

In a matter of months, I would return home from South Dakota, spend the summer in my hometown, and then transfer to a Wisconsin state school. Would I be able to survive living with my family for the summer? Knowing it was a temporary arrangement, and that I got to see Chris each day were the only positives to what felt like a prison sentence.

CHAPTER 42
Face the Music

For my sophomore year of college, I settled into a high-rise dorm room in Whitewater, Wisconsin. There were a few friends attending here from high school, but they had a year of relationship building on me. The girls I knew and had chummed with back in school had now met friends from other cities, and plans were being made to move out of the dorms next year into an apartment.

I felt like the odd one out, the music had ended, and I was one chair short. I tried to act like it didn't matter, but I always felt on the fringe of their group. And once again, they didn't know me. Once again, not their fault, but mine. I had built an armor around me to protect against any evidence or judgement that my family wasn't normal.

The University of Wisconsin Whitewater is called a suitcase college, with a city population of just over 12,000 at the time I attended. Most students came from bigger cities like Milwaukee, Racine, or Kenosha. Everyone arranged their classes so that their Fridays were free, then they would party on Thursday night and pack up their duffel bags in the morning, heading home for weekend jobs and significant others. On Sunday night, the oversold parking lots would flood with cars as students returned to campus.

I had worked all summer at the nursing facility and other home health care jobs before moving to Whitewater and saved enough to buy my own car. This was a huge step of autonomy for me, since I had never been permitted to use the family automobiles and always depended on Chris or friends for a ride.

Living with my parents had been stifling, but it was the only way to make enough money for the car and Fall term living expenses. There was nowhere to go in their apartment, it was hot and dark, blinds always drawn. It was as dusty and dirty as ever, with no privacy in the bathroom, no way to lock the door, and I still could never use the kitchen. I don't know why I was surprised. These were always the rules in "The Book of Dad," but I think returning after being away made the conditions all that more obvious.

The most disappointing and undeniable change was that Dad had gotten worse. Whatever we were pretending this wasn't, it was. He held on to the walls when he staggered around the apartment. His face grimaced uncontrollably, eyebrows raised up, eyes bugged out, then eyebrows back down and eyes squinted shut. His speech was almost unintelligible at times, and I had to listen close to hear him, but I usually didn't want to hear whatever angry nonsense he was mumbling. He still slept the day away and was up all night, and the arguing between he and my mom seemed worse than ever. How startling it was to reenter this dysfunctional chaos.

The cup half full was the distance. I was now only an hour and a half away from my hometown, and each weekend that he was available, Chris would come home from Stevens Point. The difference being that when Chris came home, he brought his dirty laundry, which his mom washed and folded and put back in a basket for him. He ate pizza and watched movies with his family. He went hunting and fishing, and on Sundays, she packed him up with Tupperware containers of hot dish leftovers and rice crispy bars to take back to campus.

When I came home for the weekend, I would enter our suffocating 2-bedroom apartment, which had seemingly shrunk in size. After I left for school my freshman year, my mom converted her daughters' shared bedroom into her own personal respite away from my father. She had bookshelves, a writing desk, and a small bed. I can't blame her, but once again, a game of musical chairs and I came up short, no room for me.

It was crystal clear when I came home each weekend that Dad didn't want me there. My mom enjoyed catching up, but

Dad seemed jealous. Many nights I found myself once again waiting on "The Green" for her to come home from work, the Deja Vu not lost on me, hoping for a few minutes alone with her before my presence poked the bear.

I had quit the nursing home but kept my home health job in town, which was a drop in my bucket of bills, but better than nothing. Doing laundry at my house was out of the question, but I could sleep there for free, and I could scarf a little food from their kitchen on the way back to Whitewater.

Was seeing Chris on the weekends worth this? As much as I tried to remain inconspicuous, each time I came home our arguments would escalate. Finally, in the heat of anger one weekend, Dad broke.

"Your mom and I don't fight when you're not here. You show up, and all hell breaks loose. Maybe you ought to stay at that fancy school of yours, and not come back around here so much," he said.

"But Dad, I have to work," I said.

"You need to stay out. I see your face next weekend, I'm gonna change the locks," he announced.

I was homeless. I was embarrassed and ashamed. What self-sufficient, straight-A kid had parents who kicked them out? I pretended it wasn't a big deal, got a job in Whitewater, and joined the minority of students who stayed on campus for the weekends. But it was a big deal, and it hurt.

My junior year I moved into an apartment with some of the fringe friends and continued my double life. To them I was a partying yet studious girl who had a steady boyfriend, when in reality I was a girl whose family was crumbling and lived each day paranoid of inheriting a fatal genetic disease.

We alternated weekends, either I drove my new car to Stevens Point to see Chris, or he drove his parents' car to Whitewater to see me. We maintained the long-distance relationship, and it felt like we might make it and be together forever. It also felt a bit like playing house.

CHAPTER 43
What We Are Getting Into

Now whenever I came home on a rare weekend, Chris's parents let me stay at their house, because he told them how difficult it was for me at mine. Of course, it was separate bedrooms for us because there would be no shenanigans. One warm spring Sunday afternoon, we had just gotten home from church with his family, and I was headed back to campus, but Chris convinced me to take a short drive first.

We wound through some country roads, listening to the radio, and then he eventually pulled into a park just outside of town and stopped the engine. We looked at the trees and sat quietly for a few minutes. He nervously fidgeted and started talking about our upcoming camping trip.

"Where should we go? Why don't you open the glove box and get the map?" He smiled at me with his classic mischievous grin.

As I reached for the compartment handle, it hit me. Chris always hid treats in my glove box for me to find later, packs of gum, special notes, and even small presents. Could this be it? I cracked the lid and peeked inside to find a square velvet box.

"Well, open it up," he said, barely containing his excitement.

I undid the ribbon and eased open the box, finding a sparkling diamond inside that took my breath away. Our eyes met. Freshman year, when it seemed we were but children, he had already asked, and I had already said yes, so no words were required. We smiled, and I slipped on the ring, making it official.

"Where should we go, who should we show first?" he asked, giddy.

I gulped. I hadn't seen much of Dad since he booted me. "Let's go see my dad."

We drove across town and found Dad in the driveway, fishing around in the back of his van. When he saw us pull in, he slammed the doors and shuffled over.

"Dad, we have something to show you," I said holding out my hand.

He took my hand, turning it this way and that, eyes squinting as the diamond caught rays of sunshine. He wasn't a traditional man, but would he have expected Chris to ask permission? I anxiously watched as the two men sized each other up.

They made eye contact for the longest time, and then Dad broke into a grin, and they shook each other's hands with a firm grip, Dad clapping Chris on the back.

"Well, we better go, we have some other people to tell," I said.

Dad waved us goodbye as we pulled out of the driveway. It had never been that easy, and I dared not think any further than this moment.

We spent the afternoon sharing our news. The rest of our family congratulated us, and hours later than I had originally anticipated, I headed back to campus. I took the backroads, County KK to Highway 11, through Juda and Brodhead and couldn't help watching the ring sparkle in the side mirror as I rested my arm on the open window.

As I drove I thought about what Chris told me before I left. A few weeks ago, once she learned of his plan to propose, Chris's mom had sat him down and asked him a pointed question.

"Are you sure you know what you're getting into?" She asked.

She then reminded him that each night she cared for Luanne, bedridden at the nursing home. Did he realize that Luanne had Huntington's disease, she would never get better, and that this disease was hereditary? She thought by looking at my dad that he had it too. Did Chris truly know the risks?

"I do know, and I'd rather have any time that I can have with her than all the time without her," Chris said.

Chris shared that his mom then said that was all she needed to hear, and they wouldn't speak any more of it. Then she lent him the money to buy this beautiful ring.

Looking back, I respect her concern. If it were my child, I would have sat them down too. Did we really know what we were getting into? Likely not.

CHAPTER 44
Checkmate

"Lori, your dad's here." Chris found me in the backyard on the deck, talking to friends of the family. His eyes were wide with surprise, and his look communicated, "Will you be okay with this?" I gave a small nod and came around to see for myself, as a queasy feeling crept into my stomach.

Dad stood in the front yard, dressed in his typical outfit of sweatpants and a faded navy-blue T-shirt, under the pretense of leaning casually against a tree, yet depending on that lean to keep his balance. His right arm swayed in an uncontrollable circular motion, which he offset with an occasional swipe at his hair, as if to smooth it back, years of that repeated habitual gesture mingled with his chorea.

My insides filled with joy and shame, swirling as oil and water in the same flask. I couldn't believe he showed to my college graduation party. I never thought he would come, yet here he was, standing on 13ᵗʰ Street for God and everyone to drive by and stare. I wanted to crawl into a manhole and close the lid. Everyone would think he was drunk or on drugs, staggering around out there.

The raised roots from the oak offered an opportunity to trip any which way he turned. I instinctively reached out and offered my arm for support, then instantly regretted that I had as he gripped hold, his weight bearing down on me. He was uncomfortably close, hugging and squeezing me. My father was proud, and I was squirming.

We held my graduation party at Chris's parents' house. There was no way I could have had it at mine. Mom told family and friends that there wasn't room at our place for all the guests, and that was the truth to be sure. We never could have had all these people, but even more so Dad might have freaked at the last second or not have gotten dressed. Company coupled with celebrations was a recipe for disaster. When Chris's parents offered to host the gathering on their backyard deck, my mother and I humbly and gratefully accepted.

Dad's voice was quiet under the steady traffic going by. "So, you're all smart and graduated college now, are you?" he asked, smiling, but the seriousness shadowed the joke.

"Yeah, I guess." I shrugged and downplayed it, as I had minimized all my previous achievements for him.

"Guess you're smarter than your 'Old Man' now, but then again you always were." He teased again, but this conversation was starting to make me nervous.

My memories travelled back to when he taught me to play chess, and I wondered if he was remembering the same time. One night when I was just nine years old, Dad dramatically retrieved the chess board from its cupboard, smoothing the box top and carefully removing the lid. We examined the pieces, my fingers running over the intricate carvings on the bishop and the knight. My favorite was the queen with her spiky crown, because she was beautiful and scary at the same time.

He hesitated at first and sized me up, as if weighing whether I was ready or even capable of learning this game. I held my breath through this long pause, hoping he wouldn't change his mind. Finally determining me worthy, we laid them out, black and white, pawns and royalty, and the lessons began.

Each night, we faced off at the coffee table. He would smile, amused as I walked into precarious plays or potential check time after time.

"Are you sure you want to do that?" he'd ask and give me the chance to take it back. After a while, he stopped offering the grace of "take-backs," and the self-professed high school dropout who couldn't read, beat me soundly each and every game. But I was gaining on him. Through several weeks of hopeless check mates, I began to put some strategy under my belt.

"Check," I said nonchalantly one evening and tried to hide the exhilaration that I felt. My heart was pounding as he methodically analyzed the situation.

After what seemed like hours, not minutes, he made a half-smile and surrendered his king. "Okay, you got me."

We unceremoniously put the pieces away, and as the lid closed on the box, my initial excitement faded. That closure felt more final than the end of any other game.

I was right. We never played again.

Even when I casually asked, "So, Dad, a game of chess tonight?" his answer was always the same, "Nope, you beat me, we're done."

Chris's father came around front to say hello. As they shook hands and began to talk, I thankfully slipped out of Dad's grip and disappeared. Normally I would have stayed to mediate or translate my father's pressured speech, but today I didn't have it in me.

I had landed a job three hours north, a real, corporate position. My dream of getting out and up would finally begin to be realized, and as thrilled as I was to fly away from this craziness, I couldn't help wondering if this was checkmate all over again. Would my ascension sever something? If I said, "So, Dad, how about a visit?" would his reply be, "Nope, you beat me, we're done."

CHAPTER 45
Wedding Day and Little Victories

"Please God, just let him hold still."

I repeated this prayer over and over, as if the repetition would increase its strength. I looked in the mirror and adjusted my veil one last time. My heart was pounding, and I tried not to envision the worst. That my dad, in front of two hundred people, was going to shake, convulse, or tip over and cause a scene. Or, worse yet, get pissed at someone or about something and begin yelling and swearing, then storm out.

I carefully ascended the steps from the basement of the church, holding onto my train, and waited in the foyer as the bridesmaids made their entrances on the arms of the groomsmen. My sister stood next to me and smiled encouragingly. As matron of honor, she was the last one to go. I looked down at my bouquet. The roses were quivering, but it was my hands underneath that were trembling. Would it be me, shaking and causing a scene at my own wedding?

I heard the beginning bars, the faint strains of "Canon in D." Here we go. I began my trek down the aisle, with an ocean of smiling faces fixed upon me. The congregation had risen and turned in one full motion. Everyone was staring at me.

I had elected to walk down this aisle alone, just one of many solo journeys I had made this far in my life. Most young brides are escorted by their father, some by both parents, others by a brother or a close relative in the absence of a father. To say that I was absent of a father was the understatement of a lifetime.

Up until yesterday, he claimed upside and down that he wasn't even coming. He said churches gave him the "Heebie Jeebies," and he might consider showing up at the reception, but no way in hell was he strapping on a "monkey suit."

The nightmare of my sister's wedding seven years ago still rang fresh. Dad, Mom, and I drove eight hours to South Dakota where the wedding was to be held, in the groom's hometown. Dad almost turned around twice because of busy highways and other motorists who had just learned to drive yesterday.

The morning of my sister's big day found my mom and me in a hotel room, bribing, threatening, and cajoling my father into his tuxedo. All three of us were in tears at one point until we finally got that man dressed and out the door. His caving words were "never again," and he spent the next several years reliving the horrors of it all and informing me that I would be eloping when it was my turn.

I felt woozy and swayed a little to one side, before I realized and righted myself. Now I knew why you take someone with you, there's nothing to hold onto out here. Must focus. There was my groom, standing what seemed like a mile away. I kept my eyes planted on that beaming light at the end of the tunnel, putting one foot in front of the other until I reached the front of the church.

My father and mother had been seated in the first row and now stood waiting for me. Dad had complied, and I was glad not to know the details. He was handsome in his black tuxedo, all of the buttons and cufflinks secured in the right places, and his bowtie cinched tightly at his neck. With his hair combed back and a big smile on his face, he looked almost like a textbook proud father of a bride.

Dad shifted back and forth with what any stranger might take for nervous energy, but what I knew was his chorea, his motions intensified by the pressure of standing in front of all these people. I brimmed with gratitude that he would go through all of this for me, to not screw up my wedding day, while another part of me was equally indignant. Any other normal father would be here, why did I have to feel grateful? But now wasn't the time for pondering the legitimacy of my appreciation.

Dad held my arm, and I could feel him tensing.

"Who gives this woman in marriage to this man?" the officiant asked.

My father answered in a barely audible whisper, "Her mother and I do."

He did it. He nailed his line.

My vows would be a piece of cake compared to making it through this. Now, he just had to let me go. Dad held on to my arm, lingered, as I turned towards the steps of the altar. Could I break from my past and move towards my future? What if, with all my strength I tried, but my past followed me? I could gently slip from my father's grip, but he was still part of me. Would his shaking movements follow me into my new life?

Dad let go, and I went up. Promises were made, rings exchanged, a kiss, and the rest was a blur of congratulations and hugs. I lost sight of Dad for most of the evening until, later at the reception, he reappeared just as he originally said he would, changed into sweatpants and a T-shirt, and looking much more like himself.

There would be no father of the bride dance for me, and no, it wasn't fair, but it could have been worse. He was here and happy for me, and we had made it through. This wasn't about luxury, it was about survival, and when you are surviving, every little victory counts.

CHAPTER 46
Best Day After

When people are asked to describe their best day ever, they respond with a variety of answers. Maybe it was the day they fell in love or the day they landed that corporate promotion. They got the leading role, earned their master's degree, or a baby was born. Invariably, the answers include their wedding day. It is probably one of the most popular answers.

My best day ever would be, not the day of my wedding, but rather the day after. The day following the big event is when the jitters have subsided, the camera bulbs have ceased flashing, and the couple takes their first steps into forever, a quiet arm and arm beginning.

The morning following our wedding night, we sat at the Perkin's restaurant on the east side of Madison, Wisconsin, having breakfast before embarking on a 3-day honeymoon to the

Upper Peninsula of Michigan. The huge American flag raised out front, trademark of Perkin's restaurants, seemed to wave for us alone, as if to announce: these people right here, in this vinyl booth, these people get a fresh start, and it begins today.

We ordered eggs over-easy with toast and bacon. Chris likes to spread grape jelly on everything, and I watched him in amusement. I tried to stop glancing over my shoulder, did my best to quell the anxious thoughts that threatened to invade my overwhelming happiness. I half expected uniformed enforcements to come bursting through the double doors at any minute and put an end to this new beginning before it even got started.

"I love you," he said.

I turned my watchful eyes from the entrance and gazed into his.

"Me too," I said and smiled back at him. This unconditional man, who took me as I was, seemed like a gift beyond opening. If I considered it too long, I would cry, so I joked instead.

"You want some eggs with that jelly?" I asked, and he smiled.

We finished our plates, and I drank the last of my coffee.

"Let's get outta here," he stretched and grabbed the check.

In the car, we cracked open the card box, which I had

nabbed under my arm as we dodged bird seed and fled the reception last night. We spent the five-hour drive to Michigan opening cards, reading the sentiments, and pocketing the cash. We were rich!

Better than any cardboard container of money was this unfolding future. As our little car wended through the winding roads of northern Michigan, we took in the autumnal display, the blaze of reds, oranges and yellows that encore the season.

Fall is traditionally the end, the dying, but not that day. Each leaf that floated to the earth was one less weight, a flotation device to grab onto. I became lighter and lighter, until I was sure I could fly to the branches and trade places with the departing foliage.

I peeked over at Chris, shades covering his eyes, one arm slung casually on the wheel, the other fiddling with the radio dial. Would he be able to live up to my desperate expectations? Would I get sick? Would he wish he had never signed up for this? I dared not wonder and just enjoy the time we would have, however long it might last. Whatever our allotment of this happiness and peace, I would always consider this the best day, the beginning.

CHAPTER 47
New Chapters and Package Deals

My husband and I moved into a little duplex on the south side of Neenah, Wisconsin, our first place together. We were renting, but this was home.

He held the painting, a wedding gift, while I poised with the hammer in mid-air.

"Go ahead then," he said.

"I'm going," I said, but then stalled and choked up.

How to tell this man, who had seen glimpses of my world in our years before marriage, but not nearly all of it. Pounding nails into a wall set my heart pounding, as if it was going to come out of my chest, and I felt light-headed on the ladder.

Putting holes in walls was clearly an infraction in the "Book of Dad," and making noise by pounding on a wall was also up there on the list. I felt like a kid out past curfew, looking over my shoulder for the city police.

Chris must have intuited because he knew me so well.

"You can do anything you want now. Whack that nail!" he said encouragingly.

And I did. I'd like to say I drove it home, but it was a bit of a flop, and Chris had to correct my attempt. After he'd set the nail properly, we aligned the frame, and stood back to admire our work. I giggled, both in relief of having gotten away with hanging a picture, and at the subject of the artwork itself.

Our best man gave us this wedding gift, a twenty-by-thirty rendition of Jesus in his best stereotypical form, with Anglo-Saxon colored skin, silky flowing hair, and a killer "come follow me" grin. He was decked out in white robes, gripping a staff, and holding an innocent-looking lamb in one arm. We were confident that his mother helped him buy it for us, and we blasphemously named the painting "Sexy Jesus." In the following years that we led youth groups, held Bible studies, and invited friends over to our home, everyone would joke about the painting and ask, "How you doin?" in true Joey Tribbiani fashion. I would laugh and kid with them, but then become nostalgic, remembering the combined terror and freedom of that first nail.

Our first years as newlyweds were filled with new friends and carefree adventures. We joined a local church, took canoe trips, played in volleyball leagues, and had a real Christmas tree that was ten feet high. Chris finished his final year of college while I started my first professional job as a technology instructor.

I was on a mission, to try and do everything that had formerly been forbidden, attempting to soften over twenty years of rigid rules and my propensity to anticipate and prevent conflict. We navigated my anxiety, as broken glass, raised voices, or any type of tension sent me over the edge. I also battled poor body image and pervasive shame at either of us being seen without clothing, which caused a constant struggle in our intimate relationship. We took one day at a time, but Chris absorbed the brunt of much of my baggage.

Always lurking in the back of my mind was my family and my genetic risk, although I avoided seeing them or thinking about it. It became tricky. Chris was close to his family, and I loved them too, and although we wanted to visit, it was a complicated package deal.

Since we both came from the same small town, it was hard to visit them and not see mine as well. I also couldn't come home without stopping by Grandpa and Grandma's. They seemed to have a sixth sense and knew whenever we were down the street, and soon my in-laws' land line would be ringing, and my grandparents would be asking, more like demanding, for us to stop over. It became so stressful that I pressured Chris to stay away more than he wanted to. I was not equipped with bravery or boundaries and so went into hiding, and my regret today is that we alienated much of our family in the process.

While I was starting my new chapter, the medical community made a groundbreaking discovery by identifying the gene that causes HD. In March 1993, scientists identified the gene responsible for Huntington's disease, pinpointing it to chromosome number 4 and naming it HTT/huntingtin. They discovered the culprit for the gene mutation, an expanded CAG repeat.

The HD gene has a trinucleotide repeat sequence of cytosine (C), adenine (A), and guanine (G.) In people without HD, the number of repeats on their chromosome is between 10 and 35, but when the number of repeats exceeds this range, a person will develop HD. The research also showed a higher number of CAG repeats equates to an earlier onset with increased severity in symptoms.

Once the HTT gene and the specific CAG repeat expansion associated with HD were identified, it became possible to develop a diagnostic test. This test could identify individuals carrying the mutated gene before they became symptomatic.

My grandmother subscribed to the HDSA newsletter to keep updated on research progress, and she was excited to share these developments with me and anyone else in the family who would listen. This should have been good news for me, one step closer to a predictive test, treatments, even a cure, but I saw it as a threat. It only added more weight to the already almost unbearable mass in my chest. Not a day went by that I didn't second guess myself for tripping or dropping something. I mentally planned for the day when I started showing symptoms and flip flopped between getting tested and chickening out.

Grandma said she was making her appointment as soon as the test became available, and then we'd know for sure whether she had HD. I knew my father would flat-out refuse, so then what? I would need to undergo testing myself to get a definitive answer, and the prospect of that was horrifying. I felt a stopwatch clicking, and the race was on, how much life could I live before this became real?

CHAPTER 48
More Than a Social Call

"Your grandma wants to see you."

Mom's voice came over the telephone line at Chris's parents' house, and I felt my stomach sinking with her words.

"What does she want?" I asked.

"She wants to talk to you. It sounds serious, so since you're here this weekend, you need to go and see her."

Mom had ventured I might be reachable at my in-laws' landline, but she seldom knew if we were in town anymore, since I usually avoided stopping by.

"Alright, I'll go over before we leave," I said.

Chris and I had traveled home because a group of friends from high school were getting together, but this wasn't how I planned on ending the weekend.

I walked the short block from my in-laws' house down

to Grandpa and Grandma's. Grandpa was out puttering in his garage, and I stepped in the side door. I gave him a hug and breathed in the scent of his machine oil and coveralls. He looked older and weary.

"We don't see you very much anymore," he said, offering a smile but still calling me out.

"It's been busy," I said, but felt guilty for not making the time.

"Go on in and see your grandmother, she's waiting for you," he said, so I climbed the porch steps and rapped on the door. There was no answer, so I popped my head in.

"Grandma, I'm here," I said. Still no answer, so I came all the way in and called louder for her.

"I'll be right out," she said.

Eventually she appeared, weaving her way from her bedroom and through the maze of antiques and memorabilia that covered every available surface of their tiny living room. She had already been moving slow, but absence makes the reality starker, and I hadn't noticed her walking this hunched over and unsteady before. In recent years, her hands had gnarled with arthritis, but now they trembled as well.

She shuffled over to the coffee table and picked up a manilla envelope with my name on it, pinching it between the thumb of one hand and the palm of the other.

"Let's go sit down in the kitchen," she said.

This was formal, not something we ever did. We always sat in the living room, her on a low-profile swivel rocker, and me perched on the white couch, which was always covered with a protector, but I did as she asked and pulled out a chair in the kitchen. There was only room for one at her table, so I sat, and she hovered above me, swaying back and forth. She opened the folder and looked me in the eye.

"Lori, I have some news for you, and I want to explain some things," she began.

Her voice came, halting. Her speech was pressured and a little garbled. How had I not noticed this before? My pulse quickened.

"Your Great Aunt May and I went to the University of Wisconsin Madison a couple months ago and got tested for Huntington's disease," she said.

My heart sank. Here we go. She had been hinting about having Huntington's disease for as long as I could remember, and claimed she would be the first one to sign up when a test became available. But my grandma was fine. She didn't look a bit like Luanne or Eilene, and I had held on to that visual comparison for the past few years, knowing full well that physical similarity had nothing to do with genetic code, and that symptom progression could vary widely between affected individuals.

Grandma not showing symptoms like her sisters was my last thread of hope that what was affecting Dad was not also

Huntington's. If Grandma was positive, that put him one step closer on the assembly line of tragedy. This was denial at its greatest level, but at the time, all I could do was hold on to that possibility, willing to accept whatever my dad had wrong with him, as long as it wasn't HD.

I didn't say a word, and she pressed on. She opened the folder and showed me a pedigree chart starting with my Great-Great-Grandfather. The print-out diagrammed six generations of our family, squares for males, circles for females, with diagonal slashes through those individuals who had since passed away. An alarming number of people produced a polka dot pattern across the page with darkened symbols, indicating they had displayed signs of HD. Signs previously determined by other family members or doctors, nothing precise. Until now, now there was a test.

"The wonderful news is that May tested negative," Grandma said. "But I tested positive. I have Huntington's disease."

Two sisters had walked into the Waisman Center together but came out forever separated by one strand of genetic code. It wasn't fair.

"I'm so sorry, Grandma," was the best I could manage and keep my emotions in check.

"I know, and it's fine. I've always known. I've always known that I had this," she said resolutely, and maybe it was a relief, to finally have her suspicions confirmed. She paused and continued. "But now you must understand that your father has it too."

"We don't know for sure," I said quickly, my voice sounding contrary and childish, even to my own ears.

She eyed me, and I avoided her stare by looking back down at the chart, resenting how she had already colored his square in with her pencil. I saw in the upper left corner that we had been issued a Family Number from the research center and thought back to our secret clinic visit many years ago. Was my sister's and my blood stored somewhere? Had our bubbles already been determined, and Grandma simply hadn't filled them in yet? I didn't dare ask, but a new emotion, a hot spike of anger, rose in addition to my fear.

"He'll never get tested," I told her.

"Perhaps we can talk to him about it and persuade him, for the good of the family," she said.

I nodded my head, showing some agreement with her, if only to make her stop talking. I knew there was no way in hell that my dad was going to get poked by a needle only to be issued a death sentence for which there was no cure.

"Just because he doesn't find out doesn't mean you can't," she continued.

She had brought extra pamphlets from the center, and as she explained the specifics of the testing process, I focused on the ticking clock hanging on the wall behind her, felt my eyes soften, and floated away. Behind rushing waters and wind, I heard bits and pieces about genetic counseling, waiting periods, not having biological children, adopting, and stopping the cycle. I picked up reality again as I heard her offer to pay for my test, best to use cash, so the insurance company wouldn't be the wiser.

"I'll think about it Grandma," I said, gulping air. I needed to get out of there.

She painstakingly put each document back in the envelope and gave it to me. I held it in my hand like it was on fire, gave her a quick hug, and told her I needed to go.

I walked back to Chris's parents' house on autopilot, wanting nothing more than to collapse into his arms and have him tell me this wasn't true, but he wasn't there.

"Chris ran to pick up some snacks for you kids tonight," his mom called from the kitchen where she was chopping cheese on the wooden cutting board that pulled out from the counter. I entered the room, and she took one look at me and knew something was dreadfully wrong. There was no fooling her perceptive eyes, and I spilled out everything my grandmother had just told me. She was quiet as I talked, working the slicer and arranging the squares of cheese on a tray. Finally, she spoke.

"I'm so sorry, but it is good that she knows. You suspect your dad has it too, don't you?" she asked.

For the first time ever I admitted that yes, I thought he

might.

"Well, we are just going to have to pray about all of this. It is in God's hands, and we love you," she said, and with a final drop of the cheese cutter handle, the case was closed, right as Chris came through the back door with bags of chips and containers of dip.

Was it that simple? Could we pray for this to go away, and it would, everything working together for good to them that love God?

Chris's mother had been working at the nursing home for more than twenty years, the longest employee there, and she had cared for every resident in that facility, including originals like my Great Aunt Luanne. She had witnessed sickness and decline, and she clearly knew what my future could hold, but she chose to trust that God would care for her children, as she covered the cheese tray in plastic wrap and sent us out the door.

CHAPTER 49
The Motor Home is Coming

The grim reaper, the Pace Arrow, the geriatric traveling show made a stop in my town tonight. I flew through our newlywed duplex, shoving dirty laundry, my husband's college homework, scummy aquarium equipment, and you name it into every available closet and slammed each door. Good thing it took my grandmother an hour to extract herself from her house on wheels. It wasn't much lead time, but I took what I could get.

In the past few years, my grandparents had traveled in their motor home more than ever, gone for months at a time out west to Montana and Wyoming and as far north as Nova Scotia. They often made impromptu visits when their excursions took them within our radius, and they were parked outside the driveway as we pulled up. Had they never heard of "phone first"?

I thought of that TV jingle, but if I had known they were

coming, I wouldn't have baked a cake. I would have not been home. Anger had been cohabitating with my fear and trepidation ever since Grandma shared her test result, and it rose again like bile in my throat.

Then they were in the door, all smiles and "surprise!" Yeesh, my skin began crawling. Chris and I had gone for the weekend on a little northern getaway after a hugely busy week of work for me and university classes for him. This Sunday evening, I planned to wash laundry, unwind, have a glass of wine, and get ready for what promised to be another grueling work week ahead.

I hardly remember our conversation, just that my mouth hurt from smiling once it was over, that and my muscles were tense from trying to be still. It was my mission to sit like a normal person while visiting with my grandparents, whatever normal was. They were always watching, those two. I was convinced they were waiting for symptoms of Huntington's to reveal themselves.

I remember the conversation turned serious at one point, when they shared that Great Aunt Luanne had passed away, which was news to us. She had lived the remainder of her life in a nursing home bed, limbs writhing, and my mind instantly recollected the nights I cared for her on my evening shifts, fearing my future was being foretold before my eyes. They gave us the funeral details, but I already planned that we would be busy that day.

If I began to shake, would they carry me off to the very nursing home where she used to live, and I used to work? Would they arrange the priest to make weekly visits? Or would they say, "I told you so," and I should have gotten tested before marrying? Would they continue to remind me how adoption is a great option for those with terminal genes?

I remained as a statue. I would not give them the satisfaction of seeing me even blink or swallow.

CHAPTER 50
Ethical Considerations

Whether to have biological children or not when you are at-risk for a genetic disease is a difficult decision. In the case of Huntington's, it can be an especially complex ethical consideration given HD's autosomal dominance, meaning no carriers allowed. If you pass the gene to your child, they will exhibit symptoms.

Some parents choose not to have biological children because they don't want to pass this risk. Others choose to proceed, because they either hope that the child will be gene-negative, or they anticipate furthered research and a cure within the child's lifetime.

Sometimes religious faith plays a factor in decision-making, and families may believe in the sanctity of human life, that each child is a gift from God, regardless of any mutated gene. Medical interventions, including genetic testing of a fetus, may not align with a couple's belief system.

Today there are several options for families considering next steps, including genetic testing prior to starting a family, adoption, and pre-implantation genetic diagnosis (PGD.) PGD, used in conjunction with invitro fertilization (IVF) first became available in the early 1990's and has since evolved in its accuracy and effectiveness. In the 1990's insurance coverage for procedures like this would have varied and often been limited.

As my husband and I anticipated starting a family, PGD wasn't even on our radar, but the rudimentary HD research I had done in previous years and the newsletters Grandma sent regularly by mail were in plain sight. Everything we had learned pointed to a 50% chance that I would have HD, if, and the IF was in capital letters, my dad had HD. But who were we kidding? Denial was my best friend, but if Dad didn't have Huntington's disease, what else could it be? Something was very wrong with him, but no one talked about it, and we continued to pretend that everything was fine whenever we saw him. Our visits had become more infrequent, but each time I climbed the green steps, I noticed further decline.

I felt selfish, cornered, and pressed to live my life quickly. I reasoned that, if we could have a child before Dad was diagnosed, then I somehow wouldn't be judged. I held an inner dichotomy, extremely worried about what others would think and yet wanting desperately to have my own way. I yearned to create a beautiful family like in the TV shows I watched and the books I read as a young girl. I was mostly concerned about what my grandparents and other family members would think of our choice, as our circle of friends in our new town was unaware of my genetic risk. Looking back, I lived life in my twenties and thirties like one big countdown, and much of my behavior and decision-making revolved around beating the HD clock.

My sister and her husband lived in Michigan and had already started their family, with one biological child and another on the way. We called long distance and talked about procreation off and on, as she was the only person who knew exactly what I was going through. She also vacillated between wanting to get tested for HD and then ultimately determining not to. At one point, she reassured me that God was in control, and we should just let whatever happened, happened. In the back of my mind, this felt like a coward's choice, but I was too cowardly to challenge it. The uneasiness and indecision ate away at me, until babies and whether to have them was all I thought about.

Babies were everywhere. Our friends were starting families, some struggled with infertility and others had unplanned surprises. The sheer paradox of life was incomprehensible, that people had babies every day, not even on purpose, while Chris and I agonized over whether to allow new life into our young marriage, into a world filled with risk and potential judgment. I felt victimized and martyred and then equally selfish and whiny.

I felt resentment towards God, who was all-powerful and chose to bring life into the world. He allowed science to intervene, He sometimes collaborated with human rebellion, but our all-knowing Creator supposedly knew what He was doing.

Questions flooded my brain. Dare we procreate? What right did we have to chance a ripple effect of this illness which destroys both body and mind and stretches its far-reaching fingers to future generations? Should I take the test and then decide? Why is there so much shame and secrecy?

I began to rationalize. Grandma's positive result remained a fresh wound from which I was still reeling, but Dad wouldn't test unless he was forced. It was only if he had HD that I would officially be at risk and could potentially pass it to our children. He was surely sick with something, but was it Huntington's? He acted nothing like Grandma, and her case wasn't exactly textbook either, as she didn't even seem that sick.

I was kidding myself, but the possibility of Dad having something else was both tragic and comforting. I sensed an urgency, time was draining, and Dad would eventually be found out. If we had a baby before this all hit, then what? Would we avoid accusation or reproachful stares from the scientific community? Whose opinions was I so worried about, my family, or perhaps this future child? Would they look at me someday and ask, "Why did you do this to me?"

Every child who enters this world has an uncertain

future, after all what is risk but an uncertainty of outcome? Does a glimpse from a DNA crystal ball offer comfort? Maybe not, when the peek didn't come with a cure. The fear of judgment wasn't gone, but it had begun to dissipate, and it would take more than a risk percentage to stop me.

CHAPTER 51
No Judgement Here

Once the bride and groom finished their song, the music kicked up to a louder and faster number, and the dance floor flooded with relatives and friends.

I sensed someone approach behind me and tensed. It was Chris's dad. I had heard he wanted to talk to me, but didn't think it would happen here, at a cousin's wedding. I hadn't spoken to him specifically about this or one-on-one since revealing my grandmother's diagnosis to Chris's mom, and I guessed that was what he wanted to talk about.

I had been avoiding everyone, wracked with conscience and indecision about children and my future. I was grieving what might not be before it had even happened.

"Come, take a little stroll with me," he said.

I swallowed and turned to follow him away from the crowd of noise and celebration. We traveled past a table of hors d'oeuvres and down a hallway to the lobby of the venue where it was quieter.

"Mom told me about your grandma," he started.

I looked down at my shoes.

"Being a science teacher, I've had plenty of genetics training in my day, and I've already sensed this could be happening for a long time." He paused and waited until I met his eye.

"It can be scary, what this might mean for your future. I know you two have been worrying about whether you should start a family."

How did he know all of this? I couldn't speak, my throat was tight, and my mind raced with what he might say next. This man had been like a father to me, for what felt like my whole growing up, and I cared deeply what he thought.

I flooded with shame and guilt. Would he accuse me of trapping his son into this life? Would he order us not to have children, not to pass this dreadful stain on to the next generation?

Sensing my agitation, he turned and kept moving. I fell into step beside him. We walked side by side, not making eye contact, but then he stopped again and took my hand in his.

"I want you to know that Mom and I love you both, and whatever you decide to do about having a family, we will support you." His eyes glistened, and I knew he meant it.

He pulled me into a side hug, and we both teared up a

little.

I don't remember much after that conversation, we both returned to the reception and mingled with family and friends, but I will never forget the love and acceptance he gave me that night.

CHAPTER 52
Now That He's Here

I gave birth to our first child, a boy, in 1996. I kept my pregnancy on the down-low for as many months as possible, nervous about telling family members who were aware of our genetic history and what their reactions would be.

As hesitant as I was to tell my grandparents that we had disregarded their wishes for us to adopt, I found that once the baby was here, they embraced him with open arms. It was almost as if her warnings had never happened.

Grandpa drove Grandma to us when he arrived, shortly after I discharged from the hospital, and once again they stayed in our driveway in their motor home. I watched closely, fearing she would drop him, as her arms shifted uncontrollably. Grandma repeatedly covered him in kisses and squished him awkwardly until he spit up or squalled for me.

Life with a new baby was busy, and we rarely visited

home. We isolated ourselves within our happy little family, skipping holidays in the name of starting our own traditions.

When our little boy was nine months old we committed to return for Christmas, staying over at my in-laws and splitting time between them, my parents, and my grandparents.

As I climbed the green steps of my childhood home, it was surreal to be holding a car seat over my forearm. I found both the state of the apartment and Dad's worsening state of mind almost unbearable. Mom had cleaned up as much as I'm sure Dad would have allowed, but it was still dark, with all the shades drawn, and a thick coat of dust covered the knick-knacks and end tables.

I was on high alert the brief time we were there, anticipating an angry outburst and planning how to either prevent or react to one. My senses were heightened by the addition of a vulnerable infant to the mix.

Dad wanted to hold the baby, and I let him, but kept a constant vigil in case he stumbled or dropped him, or worse yet, became upset or agitated. He staggered around the living room and was in constant motion. The new mother in me must have mustered courage, and I told him that if he was going to hold the baby he had to sit down, and surprisingly, he complied.

The entire experience felt like a timebomb waiting to

explode, a car teetering at the edge of a cliff. Mom took pictures and hopelessly tried to hold it all together by pretending we were fine. After we left, I couldn't shake the darkness for days.

I regret that we didn't see Chris's family more during those years when our little boy was small. We missed many opportunities for spending time together and making lasting connections in order to avoid the stress of my family's worsening situation.

Most days I would easily forget the trouble back home until Mom called with an update to the saga, usually something Dad had done or said that was slowly sending her over the edge.

CHAPTER 53
A Bluff Called

Against her better judgment, Mom brought Dad to doctor after doctor. He was constantly convinced he had some ailment or another and perseverated on a variety of symptoms. He did suffer from a hiatal hernia and acid reflux, which was likely aggravated by the excessive amount of over-the-counter medicine he regularly took on an empty stomach, routinely chasing Sudafed and ibuprofen with a swig of Maalox.

There were multiple visits to the emergency room for abdominal pain, and for months my father insisted and obsessed that there was "acid shooting out of his cheek." Mom took him to the dentist, a long-time family friend. After examining my dad, the dentist pulled Mom aside, assuring her that there was no acid to be found in Dad's mouth.

"There's nothing going on medically, this is all mental,"

he told her gently but seriously, his face grave.

The dentist suggested a saline rinse, but I believe he only provided it for Dad to make him feel heard, to appease him.

My father next insisted on seeing a proctologist, for his ongoing digestive issues. Mom scheduled the appointment and went along to see this doctor, who happened to go to our church. You pretty much couldn't go anywhere or do anything in a town of that size without people knowing your business. She remembers cringing at what this man might think after meeting with my dad.

When that visit had run its course with still no diagnosis, Dad insisted on seeing Mom's migraine doctor for headaches he was experiencing. When it was time for this exam, Mom sat in the waiting room, anticipating another strike-out in Dad's quest to fix his medical problems. It was only a matter of minutes before the doctor came out to the lobby and asked her if she could step inside, a sober look on his face. She followed her doctor back through the corridor, but they didn't return to the room where Dad was.

"While this is not my specific area of expertise," the doctor began. "Your husband clearly has some serious mental health issues. While we were in the examination room, he became very agitated and threatened his own life and the lives of others. I am by law required to report it. He's going to be transported to a mental health facility for a 72-hour hold."

Mom was without words. As many times as Dad had threatened her, us, or himself, he had finally said it to someone who had to do something about it.

Everything that happened next, took place quickly. The officers entered the examination room, restrained, and escorted my father into a squad car, and transported him to Mendota Mental Health Institute in Madison. I like to think that, even though Dad had to have been afraid and unsure of what was happening, his surroundings were at least familiar. How many afternoons had we driven around those lakes in Madison? We had cruised right past that very facility on our longer day trips, the ones that were going well.

Mom called that night to tell me everything that had transpired, and she sounded tired and weak, but relieved. The house behind her was quiet, and she wasn't having to press the receiver to her ear or holler at Dad to be quiet so she could talk to me. He wasn't grabbing the phone to put in his two cents. It was surreal.

After Dad got back from his 72-hour hold, my hope was that it had knocked some sense into him. He would realize there were things he couldn't say and couldn't do. He might learn from this and get some real help from a doctor who specialized in neurology. There was also a part of me that feared in order to get real help, the quest wasn't over, and we needed to find out what was actually wrong.

Dad was diagnosed with Bipolar disorder at Mendota and released from his hold on the condition that he attend outpatient therapy with a local psychiatrist. He was also prescribed Lithium, although my confidence wasn't high that those pills wouldn't get scattered across the kitchen counter, mingled with other nonprescription medications he was taking excessively, for any and all imagined illnesses.

We were never certain that Dad actually had Bipolar as a coexisting condition to Huntington's disease or whether he had been initially misdiagnosed. Although neuropsychiatric symptoms often present well before motor symptoms do, and can include depression, irritability, obsessive-compulsive behaviors, cognitive decline, psychosis, and dementia, there is less evidence of mania in HD. A later scientific study in 2015 would cite five cases in a family of eleven affected with HD who had comorbid bipolar affective disorder.

CHAPTER 54
First and Only Visit From Dad

My dad was coming to visit this weekend. That might sound like an ordinary statement for most people to make, but those words had never come out of my mouth before, because this had never happened before.

Dad had never seen any of my dorm rooms in all four years I attended college at two different universities. He'd never hauled boxes into my first apartment or met my roommates' parents. He'd never visited the newlywed duplex Chris and I rented the first three years we were married. He hadn't come to me in over a decade, but he and Mom were traveling to Reed Street this weekend. I was sick to my stomach.

With nervous energy I scoured the bathroom and kitchen, polishing every surface. I'm not sure what possessed me to care so much, when my childhood home was dark, dusty, and claustrophobic. What would he think of our first home, a small ranch house in a quiet neighborhood? My parents had never owned a home of their own, would he think I was putting on airs?

Sunlight poured through every open window, which was how I operated these days. Would he want the shades pulled? Was it "my house-my rules", or would I retreat to my ten-year old self, and comply?

As the afternoon lengthened and my son woke from his nap, my apprehension increased. The distance from my hometown to Neenah, Wisconsin was much longer than a day trip. It could be a three plus hour drive under normal circumstances, but what if they argued and turned around, or Dad veered into traffic? I wasn't in the back seat keeping the peace and had no way to control the outcome.

I had learned from many past experiences that the best protection from disappointment was to anticipate it. As the clock ticked, I watched the road, and had almost reconciled myself to the combined let down and relief that they weren't coming after all, when I saw Mom's car roll slowly up the street and pull into the driveway.

Dad climbed out of the driver's seat, stretched, and shuffled unsteadily to the door. He stood, hands on his hips, looking around at the neighborhood while Mom hugged me.

"Well, we made it!" she said breathlessly, but her eyes communicated "barely."

I brought them in, gave them the short tour of our three-bedroom, single bathroom home, and then it was uncomfortably quiet. Thankfully, my little boy was excited to show off his room that had walls painted with bright green paint, a big-boy bed, and a Lego set. Then he was full of more energy and wanted to go outside and show Grandpa his turtle sandbox.

We all went out to the backyard and sat on the brick patio. My father was in constant motion, wiggling in the plastic lawn chair I had set out for him. He wore cutoff sweatpants, a threadbare T-shirt, and long strands of hair hung lank over his eyes. My son noticed none of these things, and I watched in amazement as Dad took the plastic shovel offered to him and bent over to dig in the sand with my little boy.

Chris returned home from his teaching job not long after, and we made it through a pizza dinner and tucked our son into bed. The rest of the evening passed without any issues or conflict. I knew Dad was up most nights, and I had no idea how this sleepover was going to go, but I settled them into our guest room and went to bed myself. Chris reassured me that everything was going to be fine, and he showed my dad how to work the TV controller in case he couldn't sleep.

I woke early, and it was too quiet. I dressed quickly, hoping Dad would still be there and hadn't wandered off somewhere. I entered the living room and saw that he had moved out to the couch during the night. He was already awake and sat up as I came in. He claimed to have slept well but said that the couch was where he was more comfortable. I'm sure he was up and down in the night, opening and closing the refrigerator door and looking out the window. Small blessings, he was wearing sweatpants and covered up with a blanket.

My parents stayed for a couple more hours in the morning and had breakfast with us. They planned to get back on the road when it was time for me to take our son to a birthday party.

Once again, Dad insisted on driving, so Mom buckled into the passenger seat, no doubt preparing herself for four hours of gripping the "Jesus Handle." We paused in the doorway, and I watched them drive away, absorbing what had just happened as if it had been a dream, until my son tugged on my hand.

"Mommy, we have to go, so there's time for a train!" he said.

We were going to my friend Lauren's house to celebrate her daughter's birthday which required crossing a series of railroad tracks by the paper mills. Lauren and I shared childcare during the week, and there were many mornings that I grumbled about "not having time for this" when the red lights flashed and the gates came down, but my child delighted in watching train cars race by his windshield.

As the car's taillights disappeared I wondered, "What did the future hold for those two?" I did not know. Huntington's disease can progress so slowly, and yet I felt the last pages of a chapter turning. Soon a diagnosis would be a mere formality. It would only be a matter of time before difficult decisions would have to be made, but I tucked away this visit like the gift that it was.

CHAPTER 55
Screening Calls

Before the days of caller identification, receiving phone calls on a landline was a crap shoot. I couldn't even predict when he would call. It could be the middle of the day, dinner hour, or late in the evening. I'd pick up without thinking, wiping my hands on a towel, or setting the baby down, and there it was.

"Lori, this is your dad," he'd open.

Then the dread would pour in like a wave crashing the shore and dripping slowly off the rocks. I would feel instantly guilty and try to start off positive.

"Hi Dad, how are you?" I would attempt to ask breezily.

He wouldn't wait for this greeting or respond to the question and, depending on his mood, just launched in, either with an exciting play by play detail of his day or with an angry rendition of how wrong things were. Dad's words were soft and muffled, often completely unintelligible and masked with noisy breathing and verbal tics with his tongue. Agitation increased the slur of his words to the point that I couldn't make out any of them.

As the phone call ran its course, his sentences would run together. I didn't try to get a word in unless he paused, his voice lilted upwards into a question, and then I would hum a response, and he'd take right off again.

His stories could go on for upwards of an hour, and when you are attached by a cord to the kitchen wall, you soon run out of things to do. It was a long cord, and yet I'd often scrubbed all the dishes, dried them, and put them away. I chopped fruit, swept the floor, and he'd still be going. Sometimes I had to hang up.

"Dad, I really have to go," I would say.

I would try that several times before raising my voice in anger saying, "Goodbye Dad!" and clicking off. Sometimes he would call right back, sometimes I'd pick back up, and sometimes I'd stare at the phone and watch it ring until it stopped.

According to The Mayo Clinic, among the many cognitive impairments associated with Huntington's is perseveration, which is the tendency to get stuck on a thought, behavior, or action. Some individuals with HD experience obsessive or compulsive behavior, but an obsession with making phone calls is not a hallmark characteristic. Dad was diagnosed with coexisting mental health issues throughout his life, at one point bipolar and then later with schizophrenia. *Understanding Behavior in Huntington's Disease: A Guide for Professionals*, by Arik C. Johnson, PsyD and Jane S. Paulsen, PhD, explains that perseveration occurs when there is damage to the frontal lobes or the neuronal circuitry connecting the lobes to the basal ganglia. It remains a mystery whether my dad truly had coexisting issues or if all his behaviors were a result of HD.

CHAPTER 56
Creamed Cucumbers

One day I called him.

It was late summer, and my three-year-old and I had picked the vegetables from the garden. He had hauled out tomatoes, butternut squash and cucumbers all by himself in his little toy wagon. He wore his denim bib overalls and stuck his hands in the mud up to his elbows. The dog followed everywhere he went, and both paws and bare feet left black prints throughout the kitchen.

I marveled at how a child could get so dirty and not be in trouble. Tears formed in the corners of my eyes as I rewrote history, and they trickled down my cheeks. My son looked at me, a small wrinkle forming in his brow, wondering why Mommy was sad. I smiled and scooped him up in a hug so tight that he wiggled to be let go.

I wanted to do something with all this produce, and I

remembered the best tasting sweet, creamed cucumbers that my dad used to make. On a crazy whim I decided, "I'm just going to call him up and ask how he did that, like a normal daughter would."

The phone rang and rang, and I almost chickened out and hung up, but then he finally answered. Dad was confused and a little groggy. It took a minute to get through to him who I was, and then, before he could take over the conversation, I quickly asked.

"Dad, do you remember those creamed cucumbers you used to make?"

He was quiet for a minute and then, "the sour ones or the sweet?" he asked.

"The sweet ones, Dad," I said. "Could you tell me how you used to make those?"

He was quiet again, and I almost thought he was going to call me on it, on the fact that I hadn't ever sought him out for anything. Twenty-nine years old and not once ever. But he was just thinking, forming the words in his mind before they came out of his mouth.

"Well, you stir a little mayonnaise in a bowl with some sugar, you stir it good with a fork," he began quietly. For the first time I found myself pressing my ear to the receiver to hear him better.

"Then, a little milk," he said.

I received no exact measurements, but I didn't need any. I listened carefully to his pressured speech, because now as he was starting to get into it, his words came faster than he could roll them out.

I detected something else in the "pinch of vinegar" and the "refrigerate overnight." I picked out pride. The call went on a bit more, and once I had learned all I needed to know, I wasn't sure how to end the conversation.

"Well, Dad, I'm going to go give this a try, okay?" I said.

I prayed we wouldn't have to ruin this good talk with my hanging up the call to end it.

It had never been that easy. To my amazement, Dad said, "Okay, you let me know how they turn out."

With a few more goodbyes, he was off the line, but no more than the usual Midwestern farewells that linger, that Wisconsinites and Minnesotans are known for.

I served those creamed cucumbers at family gatherings and for dinner with friends often after that day. When complimented, I liked to say casually, "It's an old recipe of my dad's. He was an excellent cook, you know." I'd say it like it was the most natural thing in the world, it sounded so normal and solid coming off my tongue. I held onto that for all it was worth.

Overtaking the façade of ordinary and isolated incidents of civil conversation, Dad's phone calls escalated to an unbelievable level in 1999. He called at all hours of the night, and I wasn't getting any sleep anyway with a second new baby in the house. I was so tired from nursing at night, and with the constant ringing of the phone, it all became a blur. I began to stop answering all together. It was so easy to do.

One day I stood numbly and looked at the handset, ringing and ringing, and I watched and waited until it stopped. We didn't have an answering machine, so at first it bothered me that I didn't know who had called. After a while, I no longer cared.

CHAPTER 57
Seven Degrees of Separation

"This is going to sound crazy, but I think I talked to your dad last night."

Lauren buried her head back into her minivan and navigated the straps of her daughter's car seat. She pulled her little girl out and hoisted her to a hip, then looked at me, wide eyed and incredulous.

"Can you believe it?" she asked in her husky voice.

"Well, I don't know. What do you mean?" I stammered.

"So, here's what happened. The phone rang last night, and I picked it up. This older guy was talking really low and kind of mumbly, and he said, 'Is this Lauren? My daughter?' At least that's what I thought, so I said, 'Well, I, yeah. Dad, is that you?'"

She shifted her daughter in her arms and continued the story.

"And then he began talking, and it was rapid and hard to

understand, really pressured speech, you know what I mean? I started to get the feeling that he thought I was someone else, so I interrupted him when I could get a word in edgewise and said, 'Are you sure you're looking for Lauren? This is Lauren.'"

"And I swear I heard him say back, 'Lori? Lori, this is your dad.' And then I got to thinking, is this crazy? Could it be Lori's dad? I've gotten your calls before, as you know how our phone numbers are so close."

She was right, and I had gotten phone calls in the past that were intended for her as well. My dear friend, who lived across town and shared childcare with me, had a landline that ended in "7585" while ours was "5785", 2 digits reversed from being an exact match. We always joked about getting each other's phone calls, and with our names also being as close as they were, it's no wonder that callers could be confused if they misdialed.

But then my stomach dropped. I heard what she said. The man was mumbling, talking fast, not making a lot of sense. And he claimed to be my father. I knew what would come next.

"Lori, was that really your dad? Is he not feeling well? Is he ill?" she asked.

Lauren was a speech pathologist. She didn't just pick up on rapid speech and garbled pronunciation coincidentally, it was her specialty. She worked in a long-term care home and treated patients regularly, those affected by stroke, dementia, maybe even HD. She knew something was up, and I couldn't hide it from her.

"Why don't you come on in?" I said and motioned for the door. She followed me inside and set her daughter down, who toddled off quickly to find her playmate, delighted to see him and whatever train track or Legos he had set out for them to play with.

I knew she only had a minute before it was time for her to run to see her first patient, so I kept it short.

"My grandmother has Huntington's disease," I started, and there I stalled. I didn't know what else to say or how to put it into words. Saying it out loud somehow made it true.

"Oh my gosh, Lori, I'm so, so sorry." She grabbed me with both arms, clearly acquainted with the disorder and recognizing the seriousness of the situation. "And so, you're thinking your dad has it too?"

"Well, I'm not sure. It could be any number of things," I began, but realized how unlikely that sounded even as it came out of my mouth.

She rushed to say, "Oh yes, of course, of course," seeing the sheer terror in my eyes, but I saw something in her eyes as well, unmasked thoughts of "what else could it be?"

She hugged me again and assured me that she would let me know of any future calls from my dad so that I could call him back and sort out the confusion.

After she left the gravity hit me. No matter how much

distance I put between my past and my present, my father and his risk were catching up with my future, it was gaining on me. No amount of moxie, gumption, or pulling myself up by bootstraps would bring escape if I was tied down with double strands of helix.

CHAPTER 58
Surrendering His King

Mom called.

If the phone rang at about 10:30 AM on a weekday, I could usually predict correctly that it was her. By then my dad would have gotten up and shuffled about the house, gathered his car keys and belongings, and went out the door for his daily travels.

She would have a few minutes of peace to call me and talk before she went to work, without Dad grabbing the phone or talking over her. This was the dysfunctional routine into which we had settled.

I hesitantly picked up, relieved when she said, "Hi, Lori, it's me, Mom." But something wasn't right. I could tell in her voice immediately. It was more than her usual sheer exhaustion of trying to care for a man who did not want to be cared for.

"We have a problem," she started. "Your dad got picked up by the police again yesterday."

"Oh my God, what did he do now?" I asked. I imagined an angry outburst on one of his outings, or please no, not public nakedness.

"It was his driving. He was all over the road, and the cop pulled him over and thought that he had been drinking. They hauled him out, ran him through the ringer, made him walk the line and everything."

"But he hadn't been, had he?" I asked.

"No, they could clearly see that it wasn't alcohol, but they followed him back home to make sure he got here safely. The hard part though, is that even though he didn't get a ticket, he has to re-take his driver's test to keep his license," she said.

We sat quietly, both thinking the same thing, that he would never pass.

Mom kept me updated over the next two weeks. During that time period, the paperwork for renewing Dad's driver's license sat on the kitchen table like a chess board in check. My dad would make regular rounds, circle out to pick it up, look it over, humph angrily, and toss it back down. He paced the kitchen like a caged tiger, unable to go out on his daily drive. He was pent up, frustrated, and I imagine he was ultimately afraid of the inevitable end result.

On the last day of the retake window Dad walked into the kitchen, pulled his driver's license out of his wallet, and threw it down on the counter. He knew he wouldn't pass the retest, and he would rather surrender his king than face the embarrassment of failing.

Dad without a driver's license presented a challenging but unique opportunity for my parents to spend time together. Mom began driving Dad. Under the condition that they had to get back in time for her to clock into work each afternoon, in the mornings she would run errands and bring him along. He would sit in the car while she popped into the stores, and this then expanded to some travels out and about. They would do a few country roads, get him a coffee or a snack from a gas station, and then she'd drop him back home and go to work.

On Saturdays, if she didn't have plans, they would do a longer day trip. I wondered what it was like, them out on the road together, seeing things. A part of me felt like the little girl in the back seat again. Who would be there to ease the conversation or crack a joke? Maybe they'd be alright without me.

CHAPTER 59
A Postcard Eliminating Variables

Mom and Dad settled into a routine. She drove him to his outpatient appointments with the psychiatrist, which he treated like a penance for bad behavior, but still grudgingly agreed to go.

He saw several different specialists during this time, and I imagine they regularly consulted with one another on his case. At one point a colleague of his primary doctor, who had experience with neurological disorders, sent in a blood sample to have him tested for Huntington's disease.

To this day I cannot believe that they cajoled my father into providing a blood sample, and I also cannot fathom how the results were then revealed. A postcard arrived at my mom and dad's home address many weeks later. Mom said it looked tattered, like it had gone through several post office boxes before finding its way to its destination.

Printed in typewritten ink were the tests that were performed, and next to Huntington's disease was a check mark indicating "yes", that test had been run. After the check mark was typed the word "Positive."

That was it. A death sentence mailed on a four by six postcard without any phone call, pre or post genetic counseling, or kind eyes.

Mom's first inclination was to hide the card from Dad, knowing the potential for the results to upset him, but she couldn't hide it. When she showed it to him, he initially acted unsurprised.

"Big deal, I've always known this was going to happen," he said flippantly.

My father picked up the card and looked it over, then without another word he turned and took it with him to his desk in their bedroom. Mom wouldn't see that postcard again until much later, when she cleaned out her car's glove box in preparation to trade it in. There was the results card, with creases and lines indicating it had been folded and unfolded many times before being stashed here, by a man in the passenger seat, no longer in control of his destiny.

Mom ordered a book, which arrived in the mail, several inches thick, explaining everything there was to know at the time about Huntington's disease. She read that book cover to cover, and then she would sit with Dad and read him parts so that he could understand what was happening and what the future might hold. It was the very first time they had looked HD in the eye and begun to deal with it.

Now that he had an official diagnosis, my mom tried applying for disability for Dad. After countless forms and phone calls, she was crushed to learn that he didn't qualify, because he hadn't worked at a formal job in the past ten years. Had he gotten diagnosed earlier, their finances would have been in a much better place.

Shortly after Dad's diagnosis, he received a call from his cousin and once close friend who still lived in Colorado. Although the years and distance had separated them, they were still connected, unfortunately by a disease. His cousin had called to tell Dad that he too, had recently been diagnosed with Huntington's disease. Mom said they spoke on the phone for close to an hour, a rare exchange in which Dad paused and gave windows for his cousin to speak.

I was grateful that my parents were finally coming to terms with the situation, but this now brought me and my risk one formality closer. For all the holding out and denial I had done that Dad might have something, anything other than HD, that variable had been eliminated. He was positive, and I was officially at risk with a 50% chance of inheriting this devastating illness.

My own self judgment and shame filled me. I had ignored the advice of my grandmother and called her paranoid. I had held on to religion, claiming that God would protect us. I had thumbed my nose at fate and the future and asserted, "you only live once." I had done everything in my own selfish power to have a family, a normal happy family.

What had I done?

CHAPTER 60
Anything But a Party

Despite our hopes that Dad would take his meds and settle in with improved, more stable behavior, his moods and other physical symptoms eventually worsened. He would be up all hours of the night, staggering and pacing, ranting with the lights on, while Mom was trying to sleep before she had to go to work the next day. Their arguments reached an unbelievably escalated level.

Dad had been dutifully seeing the psychiatrist each week, and although he seemed to like the attention of being a patient, he also viewed it as probation with good behavior, and eventually became obstinate about going. He began out bursting at the doctor, and she wasn't going to put up with it. She privately talked to my mom about her options, one of them being a divorce, the other a three-party commitment.

In Wisconsin, a Three-Party Petition for involuntary

commitment is a legal document claiming that a person meets all three criteria for civil commitment for a maximum of six months: they are mentally ill or drug dependent, they are treatable, and they are considered dangerous to themselves or others. The petition must include notarized statements from three adults describing the person's dangerous or violent behavior.

It just so happened that there were three people who could attest to Dad needing care despite his unwillingness to accept it, my mom, my sister, and me. My sister and I traveled back to our hometown and met with his doctor. As she instructed, we then crafted statements backing the criteria for his commitment and had them notarized.

As we stood at the counter of a local bank, I watched the notary review our paperwork. "Does she know what this is?" I wondered. "Does this woman know that we are signing our dad's freedom away?" This is such a small town, and the banker looked familiar. "Does she recognize his last name? Does she know who we are?" Paranoia creeped in, and I jumped when her notary stamp hit the paper with a thud. We took our documents and hastily left.

My sister and I stayed at my in-law's house, not wanting our dad to suspect we were in town, and while I loved cozying with her in the spare room and catching up on each other's lives, it was anything but a party. The entire process felt secretive and under-handed.

The next day I hugged her tightly, and we said goodbye, as she would head south towards Chicago and eventually Michigan, and I would return north to Neenah.

"Hopefully this gets him the help he needs," I said.

"Yes," she agreed, "and gets Mom the break she needs."

Days later, Mom arranged to be out of the house when the police came with the court order. They served the paperwork to Dad, who initially refused to let them in. I imagined him, wrapped in a towel, peeking through the custom peephole, and cursing the cops. During this episode he made frantic phone calls and left messages for my grandmother to come and save him. Eventually the officers gained entrance and transported Dad back to Mendota, where he would wait for a court date to determine next steps.

Communication between our families had broken down since Dad could no longer drive over and see them, so Grandpa and Grandma hadn't known about the commitment plan. Grandma was outraged and called my mom at work to play her the machine recording of my father's desperate pleas. They didn't understand and were angry and afraid.

My grandmother was 20 years older than Dad and yet showed less than half of his current symptoms. Scientists had recently learned that the number of CAG repeats in the HTT gene held a key relationship to the severity of symptoms and the pace of decline of those affected by HD. One Huntington's case could look nothing like the other, even in the same family. Despite this scientific explanation of why Dad was struggling with psychiatric Huntington's symptoms more than she was, to Grandma, it felt like we were picking on her son.

A week later Mom had to go to court, where she would testify to Dad's state of mind and provide evidence to the three criteria for commitment. She called me on her flip-phone from the parking lot of our town square before going inside the courthouse. Using precious and expensive minutes, I tried to encourage her, but only had so many words.

Once she entered, she mentally readied herself to see her husband. An officer escorted him in, but she was not prepared for him to be in hand cuffs. During the proceedings he kept trying to talk to her, or anyone else who would listen, and was repeatedly shushed by the judge.

The judge knew my dad and called him by his first name. I stopped being surprised a long time ago by this small community where everyone knew everyone. The judge presiding over the hearing was a former high school classmate of my parents, and Mom remembers them riding their Harley-Davidson motorcycles together around that same town square, what felt like a lifetime ago.

The evidence was presented, the judge ruled, and Dad

was committed for an extended stay at Mendota. This bought some time to get his medication regulated and to figure out what to do with him next.

CHAPTER 61
Apartment Makeover

While Dad was gone at Mendota, my mom opened every window in their house. She used the vacuum cleaner to suck a coating of dust out of each windowsill. She washed the curtains, and then she kept going. She moved all the furniture into the middle of the living room, and she repainted the walls. The walls of our upstairs apartment hadn't been painted ever, not since they had moved in over 25 years ago.

I think it was therapeutic for Mom to go through and clean out everything, wipe down counters, remove the grime. I wondered, was she removing a bit of my dad, the residue of their dysfunction with every swipe?

Several weeks later, Dad was released and came home from treatment docile and medicated. Mom went to pick him up in Madison, and for once he didn't complain about her driving. She told me that she prepped him casually on the ride back but became more and more afraid of his reaction as they got closer to home. What would he think of her efforts to make the apartment look better? I imagined her apprehension, as this makeover would surely not have been approved in the "Book of Dad," heck moving his keys off the kitchen counter brought wrath like none other.

They climbed the steps slowly and entered the house. Dad walked in and set his knapsack down, looked around, and slowly took in the bright, decluttered space.

"It looks good in here. You did a nice job," was all he said.

CHAPTER 62
Absence of a Caregiver

"I can't take it, not one day longer," Mom said, her voice strained and holding back tears of anger and desperation.

I had been listening to her on the phone for well over an hour as she ran down a list of the latest antics of Dad, his bizarre behavior, including angry outbursts and violent threats to drive his van without a license, into a wall, with her in it. He once again was refusing to take his meds, and they were strewn all over the kitchen counter. He had become completely nocturnal, sleeping all day, and then awake all night. He'd barge into my old bedroom, where Mom slept with hopes of peace and quiet, flip the light on and begin pacing back and forth and rambling disjointedly. If she complained, he would only get angrier and louder, prolonging the episode.

She was in frequent communication with his doctors and had recently contacted both Social Services and the police. She now also consulted a lawyer, and provided recordings of his aggressive behavior, but the guidance she received was limited. Dad's behavior was abusive, but she needed to leave the home or call the police each time to create a paper trail before anything else could be done. Mom was considered Dad's caregiver, and unless she left him, no one else would step in, and he would not get the care he needed.

I could tell she was at the end of her rope. We devised a plan by which she would leave their home and come and stay with us for a short period of time, to see if Social Services could step in and get my dad's care needs sorted out.

Mom was afraid of the repercussions of leaving him. Many times, during arguments, Dad made violent intimidations about finding her, hurting her, or ending both of their lives. At the time she described it, it seemed crazy. How could someone who couldn't work or drive, let alone walk down the green steps without stumbling, actually do any of those terrible things he threatened? And yet, if I channeled my 10-year-old self, I knew I would believe everything that he said. I knew that if I spent but a few days back in my childhood home, I would have believed that he could have ended my life as well.

At the same time she feared what he would do once he discovered she left, there was equal concern from all of us for how Dad would survive without her there to take care of him. He wasn't heading to a hang-gliding adventure with his buddy, and this was no road trip down country backroads. This was a defining moment for all of our futures.

The human services staff at the county assured us that they would pay a home visit after Mom left, promising they wouldn't let more than a day or two go by without making sure he was okay.

Over the next couple weeks, my mom made her plans and got her affairs in order. She quietly quit her job of 30 years at the data center, without a big celebration or retirement ceremony. In the name of Spring cleaning, she organized some of her things in their tiny apartment, taking a donation box to charity, but not so much that Dad would detect anything out of the ordinary. She went to the grocery store and stocked the fridge with everything that he liked to eat, and she pre-paid all the bills that would be coming due in the next few weeks.

Then one chilly morning in April 2000, Mom packed the essentials she had tucked aside in advance and loaded her car while he was still sleeping the morning away in his usual style. She tiptoed down the stairs and began driving north.

The telephone started ringing before she had even arrived, but I did not answer. After she got to our house, I helped her unpack and settle into the guest room. The land line rang once more, and this time I did pick up the phone.

"Is your mother there?" Dad asked without saying hello, his voice pitched with anxiety.

"Yes, Dad, she is. I'll put her on."

I listened to her side of the conversation, which was very few words intermixed with many, many of his, and when she could get a word in, she explained that she needed to leave so that he could get help. I remember her repeating multiple times that she was not a nurse and couldn't do it anymore. She told him she would be staying with me for a little while until he could get the help he needed. He insisted she was leaving him for someone else and was divorcing him.

Mom finally ended the call upset and rattled, hanging up the receiver while he was still talking. The phone immediately began ringing again, and we let it ring out. It continued to ring off and on throughout the evening. A couple of times we picked up, and she engaged him in more conversation, trying to reason with him, but it swiftly went downhill, and eventually we took the telephone off the hook.

As promised, the county Social Services agency paid my dad a visit the following day and contacted us afterward to give a report. The caseworker came up the green steps, through the inside porch, and knocked on the door. Dad eventually let her in, first cracking the door to see what she wanted, and then opening it a little bit further when he learned she was there to help, and she wasn't the police.

It only took a few glances to survey the dark apartment and see medication scattered and food spoiling on the kitchen counter. She took notes and promised to return again the following week to see if he needed anything. Over the course of three weekly visits, the situation descended into a state of disarray, my father stumbling unclothed, incoherent, and showing signs of dehydration. This was the evidence needed. In the absence of a caregiver, the system would see that my dad needed help. Whether he wanted the help or not, he would be getting it.

Mom stayed with us the rest of that year. We put our boys in bunk beds and gave her one of their bedrooms, and they thought it was one giant holiday for most of the time.

Eventually she found an apartment, a new job at a local department store, and started to work through her finances, which were an accumulated disaster after supporting a family and a disabled spouse on her own for the past 30 years.

CHAPTER 63
2.5 Children

Chris and I had agreed that we would stop at two children even before we found out that Dad was positive for Huntington's disease. It made sense, we had two sweet boys, a puppy, and a happy home. But my heart wasn't on board with this plan, and inwardly I grieved as our infant son passed through each growth stage. I packed away tiny onesies, never to be used again, and shed tears when he no longer found comfort in being swaddled like a burrito.

Looking back, I was likely facing Postpartum depression, Situational depression, or possibly a combination of both. I battled remorse for having pursued biological children while at-risk for HD and felt sorrow at choosing not to have any more. Many days getting out of bed was hard, and my oldest watched too much TV while the newborn napped, as I stared at the wall wearing days-old pajamas.

When our baby was almost 8 months old my mood swings flattened and were replaced by sickness rising in my throat.

A missed cycle. How could it be? Well, obviously I knew how it could be, but with the second one not even walking yet? In the morning I bought a test, and the plus signs didn't lie. I was pregnant again. With a mixture of anxiety and elation, I waited until Chris got home and told him the news. His wide eyes and then a big grin said it all.

"Why not? Let's bring on the chaos!"

Despite our shock and amazement, I felt a spark of life deep within me, and although I was now more tired than I thought a human could ever be, I couldn't stop smiling. I didn't care anymore what people in or outside of my family would think or say. After a month or two of weathering the morning sickness, the next time we were in our hometown, we told Chris's family.

Overall people smiled and congratulated us. I never knew whether it was genuine or filled with fear and judgement, maybe a mixture of both? Our families said they were surprised that another baby was on the way so soon rather than state we were reckless. Our friends, who knew next to nothing about my at-risk status, teased us about buying stock in diapers and playing zone versus man-to-man defense.

CHAPTER 64
18% Interest

The muggy air clung to our skin. As the first rain drops began to fall, Mom and I found a parking place and climbed out of her car.

This place was a shack, less of an office and more of a trailer, a mobile home with a handicapped ramp. "Bad Credit? No Credit? We Have an Automobile for You!" the tattered sign promised.

We stepped inside. At one hour before closing time, there was at least a dozen staff members, scurrying like stressed out squirrels from one office to another, making photocopies, talking on the phone, and clicking the keys at their computers.

Mom checked in at the front counter, and then we had a seat in the waiting area, which was basically just an arrangement of chairs in the middle of the room. I glanced around and felt a little claustrophobic. Plaid hotel room drapes hung across the windows and against the faux wood grain paneling. I watched the receptionist try Plans A, B, and C to get the copy machine to cooperate.

Finally, my mother's name was called, and she nervously took her envelope of references and her purse and followed a young girl back to one of the tiny cubicles. Mom looked like she was headed for the principal's office.

It was with mixed emotion that I had agreed to travel with my mother to this car-credit center from hell, but she needed reliable transportation for her new job. My spirit was divided between sympathy that she was in such a jam and utter resentment that she had let things get this bad.

And then, the guilt. Things were this bad because she had been taking care of me and my sister and had refused to divorce Dad no matter how ugly he had been to her in their home as his disease progressed. My wedding was probably still on a credit card somewhere at the bottom of her purse or on a desk at the collection agency. Mom had worked hard her whole life, always scraping to provide for us, and I was sliding into the caretaker role. I tried to settle in with a book but was easily distracted, as through the entrance came all walks of life.

A twenty-something with acne and a Grateful Dead T-shirt returned to the parking lot to bring in his parents who had been waiting in the car. Without a co-signer, his loan wasn't likely to go through. The parents shuffled in, the dad holding his wife's arm to guide her legal blindness to another cubicle. They answered questions about their rent and how long the father had been at his job. An interest rate was secured, and a weekly payment was arranged to be garnished from the kid's paycheck. The boy smiled appreciatively at them both, and then tried to act like he hadn't really needed them and didn't care either way how this transaction turned out.

Another couple darted in the door, soaked from the now downpour outside. They dressed to match in Green Bay Packer jerseys. It was a Monday game night in Green Bay, and they were loyal fans. Her 80's teased hair was flattened by the showers, leaving an Aqua-Net aroma floating in the air. They had test drove an older model Honda Accord, and now sat at the desk in yet another cubicle, awaiting results. Her husband looked grim, I imagined he had hoped for that Dodge pickup out there, but they were paycheck to paycheck and would take what was offered.

Ordinary people were everywhere, both hopeful and desperate at the same time. Excuses and explanations were shared at each desk, life stories of hardship and circumstances out of their control, the paper mill was laying off, medical bills have been high. The staff listened sympathetically, and in all aspects treated their customers with dignity and respect, but I wondered what was shared in the break room. Were these customers the butt of financial humor, small chuckles behind hands?

I slouched in my vinyl chair and drank nasty coffee from a Styrofoam cup, my nose in my book. Occasionally I noticed some eyes scanning my way. At first, it was just other clients whose eyes were roving the room. Their looks seemed to seek companionship, as if to ask, "are you in the same boat as me?"

"No, I'm not, thank you very much," my eyes replied, giving off a hostile message. Then, as closing time approached, staff glances started coming my direction, and eventually, one worker even paused to ask if someone had assisted me.

"I'm just waiting for my mother," I assured him, and he moved on.

My heart filled up with a haughty, prideful dose of "you've got to be kidding that I would be here on purpose," and then was immediately doused with a generous wave of empathy and shame, as I realized that God's arms were fiercely wrapped around this building and all its precious occupants.

CHAPTER 65
It's Complicated

With Mom out of the picture, Grandpa took the reins and assumed guardianship of my father. It is hard to believe he was agreeable, because if there was a social media status label at that time to describe Grandpa and Dad's relationship, it would have said "it's complicated." Over the years they had worked together, took care of Grandma together, despised each other, and now at a stage in life when most parent-child roles began to reverse, here was Grandpa, willing to become Dad's guardian.

Dad spent the first few weeks after Mom left town at Mendota, getting his medication once again regulated while the county staff figured out what to do with him. His first placement was back in our hometown at a nursing home on the outskirts of the city. There were few facilities in our area that cared for neurological disorders, and this place had a wing for dementia and Alzheimer's. This was not the same care facility where Great Aunt Luanne had lived or where my mother-in-law still worked, and for that, I was relieved. My circles were already intersecting to the point of complete overlap.

Grandpa and my dad settled into a routine in which Grandpa would go out on the weekends and pick him up, take him for a drive through some country roads and then bring him to Grandma's for dinner.

After Social Services stepped in and Dad was out of the apartment, Mom returned home to move the rest of her things out, and she boxed up Dad's coin collection, special photographs, and other memorabilia. Grandpa kept Dad's junking van and parked it at their house, storing all of Dad's memories inside, so that when he came over, he could spend time in the van, having a sense of familiarity, even though he could no longer drive it.

Grandpa told me later that the hardest part was the end of each visit, telling Dad it was time to pack up and go back to the nursing home. I don't know how many struggles they had getting him back in the car to return to the care facility, but I know that it must have been challenging. Even my grandmother became fatigued by his visits, as her own symptoms of HD crept along in their assault on her mind and body. Grandpa wasn't getting any younger, and even though he was tough as nails, I could tell the few times I was home, that caring for both of them was taking its toll.

Eventually the nursing home would state that they were not adequately staffed or equipped to handle a unique case like my dad's, and he was transferred to a group home for adults with disabilities about an hour northwest. This would be the first of many different placements, where Dad would rage about his roommates and their cognitive disabilities, and refuse to attend day program activities, which he called "school."

Our baby girl was born in 2001, and we moved into a new, bigger home in a nicer neighborhood with a sought-after school system. My days were occupied with parenting and running my technology consulting business, while Mom flourished in her apartment across town, hanging her own pictures without repercussions and experiencing the freedom I had felt since making my own exit.

With a busy young family, visits back to our hometown become more infrequent, and it was tempting to put the situation out of sight, out of mind. I found myself successfully lulled into a state of pleasant oblivion for extended periods of time, until a trigger would pull me back under like the tide.

CHAPTER 66
Backup Co-Guardians

Chris and I brought the kids back to our hometown for a rare visit with his parents the summer of 2003. As usual, we paid an obligatory visit to my grandparents who still lived down the street from Chris's childhood home. Grandma hauled out snacks, and we sat around making pleasantries for the first hour. After that, the kids were getting restless in their tiny home, so Chris walked them back to his parents' house, miraculously without my grandparents trying to persuade them to stay longer. Once Chris returned alone, Grandpa sat down and got right to business.

"Lori, my heart's not good." He looked me in the eye and gave it to me straight.

"I need to go in for surgery, and they want to do a 5-way bypass. But before I agree to going under, I have to sign off on a plan for your dad."

"I'm not sure I understand," I said.

He took a deep breath. "If I don't make it out, there has to be a plan, and I'm asking if you will take charge of him? Will you be his guardian if I don't come out of the surgery?"

"What on earth, Grandpa? You not coming out of the surgery?" I asked.

But he was serious. The look in his eye told me he wasn't so sure he was going to make it out. I looked over at Chris, and he looked back at me, but I couldn't read his expression.

"Okay, can I think about it?" I stalled.

"You need to tell me soon," Grandpa said. He took off his glasses and rubbed his face, then put them back on and told us he was scheduled for surgery in two weeks.

"I'll stop back tomorrow before we leave," I told him. Chris and I held hands and walked slowly back down the street to his parents' house talking it over.

"I just don't know if I can take on this responsibility," I said. "I can't even be in the same room with my dad without turning into a little girl!"

Then I pictured the battle Grandpa went through each time he had to coerce Dad back into the vehicle to go home after weekend visits.

"How am I going to get him back to the facility if I take him out on an outing? Wait, I don't want to take him out on an outing!" I started to panic and talk rapidly, and Chris put his hand on my arm.

"You can do this, and you will, because you're not going to do it alone. I will do it with you," he said.

"What do you mean? How can you do it with me?" I asked.

"There has to be a way that they let two people be guardians. When we go back to see your grandpa tomorrow, let's tell him we'll do it, but we're signing up to do it together. I can handle your dad, you know that."

"I can't ask you to do that," I said.

"Well, good thing you didn't ask, I volunteered," he said.

We returned to Grandpa and Grandma's house the next morning and talked through the details. Yes, there was a way to be co-guardians, and we signed on the line. I gave my grandma hugs and kisses and wished my grandpa well in his surgery. We walked slowly back to my in-laws, carrying a box of legal paperwork that Grandpa insisted we hold onto "just in case," packed up the kids, and headed north towards home.

Grandpa went into open heart surgery the following month, at University of Wisconsin Madison Hospital. He survived the operation, but a significant lack of oxygen to his brain put him into a post-operative coma. When he awakened, he was disoriented and angry. The doctors recommended that family come and see him as soon as they could.

Enter the backup quarterbacks. We were in limbo, as my

grandfather was still alive, we weren't the legal guardians on paper. But his prognosis wasn't good. As newly minted co-guardians, we should bring a son to see his father, shouldn't we? Chris and I talked it over and agreed that, even though they'd had a roller coaster relationship over the years, my dad should see his father, especially if it might be for the last time. But the logistics seemed impossible.

"Chris, if my grandpa couldn't even get my dad to go home after visiting his mother, how on earth are we going to transport him to Madison, to a University Hospital and back again?"

My mind traveled back to the day trips on the country roads and the longer day trips to the Henry Vilas Zoo. I hadn't forgotten how, if just one thing went wrong, the outing ended badly. There were so many thousand things that could go wrong on this kind of a day trip.

"Which is why you're going to let me do it, and you're not going to worry about it," he said.

"I got this." I had never seen him so resolved.

We made some phone calls to the county human services and the new group home where Dad was staying to set up the arrangements. Chris left the next day and drove south to pick him up. It felt like he was gone for days, as I waited at home, anxiously wondering just how terrible this trip could go.

Chris had a story to tell when he got back home late that

evening. I'm sure he downplayed much of it, but he also recounted his experience honestly. In what seemed like scenes from a movie Chris replayed how he managed to get my dad in our minivan. Dad wouldn't put on his seat belt, and Chris didn't fight him. My father seemed to understand where they were going and why, so he settled in as the vehicle got moving. Once they arrived at University Hospital, Chris found a valet.

"This guy needs a wheelchair," he said.

The valet hopped to attention, parked the van, and produced a wheelchair. Dad refused to ride in that "Old Man Cripple Buggy," so they set off on foot through the winding corridor maze of the UW Madison Hospital system, Dad staggering like a drunk. Yes, there were stares. Chris said everyone was eyeing them, and he was stopped twice by security guards asking if he needed assistance.

"But once I explained that he had Huntington's disease, they saw it for what it was. He wasn't drunk or high, he had a disease. There's a difference between staring at someone and recognizing a situation."

He was right, and maybe I was too close, and I had never gotten past the stigma, shame, and underlying fear of there being something wrong with him and, therefore something being wrong with me next.

"Did he talk to him?" I asked.

The ultimate question. Had this whole journey been

worth it?

"Yeah, you know he did. He touched your grandpa's hand, mumbled a few words, and for once, his 'Old Man' didn't have anything to say back. I think it was good for your dad to see him. I'm glad I took him."

Then Chris grinned and continued, "Then the best part? Once I hauled him out of there, we got back in the van and took a drive through the Arboretum. Your dad was the happiest I have seen him in a really long time, just looking around at all the trees and the water. We went super slow, and I saw his whole body relax. He even stopped talking, and just took it in."

I hugged this man. I have no idea what I did to deserve him.

"Well, honey, you did good. Sounds like one hell of a day trip, when so many things could have gone wrong," I said.

Days later we learned that Grandpa wasn't going to get better. The doctors had initially been optimistic that he would resolve the disorientation and anger, but now his body was shutting down. They released Grandpa from the UW Madison Hospital and sent him, of all places, back to the same long-term care facility in our hometown where Dad spent his first years as a ward of the state.

CHAPTER 67
Absence of Another Caregiver

Grandpa's placement in the nursing home left my grandmother home alone, and it quickly became clear how much care she needed in his absence. Her visible HD symptoms included mild chorea and some difficulty walking. She struggled to get her words out, and although she chewed and swallowed her food slowly, she was prone to choking. She didn't appear to show any advanced psychological symptoms, but my only comparison was to Dad. She was lucid and understood that her husband was seriously ill and wouldn't recover.

We left the kids with my mom and traveled back home. Grandma hadn't wanted to ride in the car to Madison to see Grandpa, but now that he was closer, she could make the trip across town. I took up the reins for this effort, loading her carefully into my vehicle, and transporting her to the nursing facility. She sat by his bedside and held his hand as tears ran down her face, and I think she knew this was the last time she would see him alive. We stayed for just a little while since she couldn't tolerate sitting up in that position for very long, and then she was ready to go.

I brought her back and got her settled in a chair. As tiny as that house was, it felt cavernous without his presence. Grandpa took up a lot of real estate wherever he went, but he was also a comfort and a caretaker for her. She asked me to do one thing before I left. I was staying at my in-law's house for the night and headed home in the morning.

"If it's not too much trouble, could you please pull off these stockings? I hate them," she said.

I'd performed the Ted Hose removal process what felt like a million times when I worked at the long-term care facility, and I quickly bent to my knees to assist. As I worked the compression socks from her legs, I realized that, although her symptoms and behaviors were milder than my dad's, she was in end-stage Huntington's. She could hardly walk, but my bigger concern was her struggle with breathing and food intake.

Pneumonia is one of the most common causes of death for those with HD, as they often aspirate their food. The harsh reality was that when my grandpa passed away, there wouldn't be anyone to take care of my grandmother. I couldn't think beyond the task at hand, anything more than that, and I was completely overwhelmed. We had already agreed to take care of one HD patient. How could we possibly take care of two? And what if there became a third, me?

The call came from my Great Aunt May in the middle of the night, telling me that Grandpa had passed away. She asked, could I go over and share the news personally with her sister?

"Of course," I told her.

It was 3:30 in the morning. I got dressed in some sweatpants and walked back down the road. I tapped lightly on the door, even though I knew Grandma wouldn't hear, and entered. She was curled up asleep on the couch, her breathing labored. I don't know if that was her original plan or if she had been having trouble getting in and out of bed these days since Grandpa hadn't been there to help her.

I sat down next to her on the couch and watched her in sleep, her body still making small movements, but she was the most still I had seen in a long time. I hated to wake her, but she must have sensed me there and been sleeping lightly, because she stirred and opened her eyes. I gave her a soft smile.

"Grandma, I came over because, Grandpa is gone. He passed away about an hour ago."

She just nodded her head, closed her eyes, and held my hand. I wondered, at this point, what do you do? Do you sit there quietly? Do you get them a glass of water? I didn't know how any of this worked. Great Aunt May had said that she was getting up and coming over from the farm, so I knew she would be here within the hour. I told Grandma that I would wait with her until her sister arrived, but no, Grandma said she would be alright. She was going to try to go back to sleep or at least rest for a little bit more until May got there, and I should go. She knew I had a long drive to get home. I squeezed her hand tight, told her I loved her, and got up to go.

Since she exhibited fewer of what are considered the more distasteful mental HD symptoms, Grandma didn't have trouble obtaining health care assistance in our county. She was able to hire visiting home health aides for a while, but then would eventually be placed in an assisted living environment. Grandma worried about her son and what would happen to him, so I assured her that he would be in good hands.

When we got home, I cracked the lid on the cardboard box Grandpa had sent with us last month to find mounds of documents, including health care bills, receipts, bank statements, and communications from the county. He had typed some letters, but other papers were completed old-school, handwritten in his slanted scrawl. I put my head in my hands.

Chris and I stepped up to become legal co-guardians. We had no experience in how to care for someone with a degenerative neurological illness, let alone the pissed off father I had grown up with, who we soon found out would detest caregivers almost as much as church.

CHAPTER 68
Panini

"Are you my guardian?"

Dad's voice came across the telephone line with crystal clarity, as if he had summoned the Earth, moon, and stars to form the words necessary to ask that one question.

"Yes, Dad, I'm your guardian," I replied.

He then launched into a muffled verbal stream, steadily increasing in agitation, pace, and volume. I picked out a word or two, including "ice cream" and "TV," and it became clear that Dad had several issues at the group home, including running out of snacks, hating his roommates, and silencing the television, which played too loudly.

Calls came like this at the most inopportune times. We would be heading out for our son's flag football game or have a house full of guests, and the phone would ring. I began to dread its sound like years past when he lived at home, the only difference now being Caller ID. But as his guardian, letting the phone ring out or taking it off the hook was no longer an option.

I inevitably picked up to a crisis, a flurry of words with jumbled speech that was impossible to understand, the gist being Dad needed medicine but wouldn't go to the doctor, there wasn't any chocolate ice cream, or there were other residents in his room. Other days he just felt that life wasn't fair, and he would ask repeatedly why his wife had left him.

I would ask Dad to pass the phone to the caregiver on duty so that we could have a conversation, and sometimes he would, but other times he would hang up on me with a burst of what I took to be swear words. When he did put the assistant on, I got mixed results. There is no way to say this without sounding stereotypical, but the usual group home caregiver we encountered was not there for the philanthropic effort, the exception being those who were pre-medical and therefore passionate about the care they provided to the residents. Most others punched the clock, because they hadn't found a way to earn a living anywhere else and sounded bored or too busy to be bothered.

Today I learned that yes, I had guessed correctly, he was out of ice cream, but the real problem was that when Dad saw it was gone, he ripped the door off the freezer. I would now be writing another check to the group home to pay for the damages.

Last month he wrenched the television off its wall mount, with what appeared to be super-human strength, because the volume was too loud. He somehow wound up breaking a window in the process.

According to the Pew Research Center, the "Sandwich Generation" refers to people who are simultaneously caring for their aging parents and their minor children. To say that I felt sandwiched at this time would be an understatement. The sociological research surrounding the "Sandwich Generation" focuses mostly on financial constraints, but finances were the least of my trouble. Dad was issued a monthly stipend from Social Security, for which we could purchase any of his personal supplies, but he wasn't allowed to gift to his grandchildren or use the money in any other way, and if his bank account breached the allowed balance, we were penalized. The cup half full was that I had plenty of funds to write checks for repairs to refrigerator doors, to purchase new television sets, and order replacement windows.

I felt the squeeze, not financially, but in the stress of balancing my family, trying to keep positive with the kids and explain why this Grandpa wasn't a part of their lives, and yet commanded so much of our time. It constricted my heart, and the utter despair of witnessing him slowly lose his dignity collided with the accumulated hurt, resentment, and shame from a lifetime with this inadequate father. It was the daily fear and paranoia that I would wind up in the very same boat. If his erratic behaviors were the result of HD, all the self-control I could muster wouldn't stop this from happening to me, would it? No, the squeeze was not a sandwich, it was better described as a Panini. I felt pressed on both sides with a hot iron and believed that any day now my insides would surely melt.

CHAPTER 69
May First and the Escape to Mendota

Perhaps I got my goalsetting mindset from Dad. My father was born on May 1, 1946, and he was obsessed with his birthday. For a man who didn't care much about any other holiday, he was convinced that all goals, deadlines, and things anticipated should be accomplished by his birthday. Over the years he would make comments like, "By May 1st, I am going to lose 30 pounds!" or "By May 1st, we're gonna get the hell out of Dodge!"

Dad carried his fixation with the first of May to each stay in what would become over half a dozen different facilities during the course of his illness. Each year that I flipped the April page I would look at the calendar and cringe, wondering what outlandish phone calls I was going to get from him or the staff on this birthday. Would he have broken more furniture, taken a swing at an aide, or refused to get dressed? I didn't visit Dad on his birthdays, but I would package up photos and some coloring pages from the kids to send to his current address and wait for the call to come.

Nothing quite topped the May 1st when Dad made his escape. He had just recently been transferred to a facility near Madison, Wisconsin, which was designed for residents with cognitive disabilities, all of whom were transported by van to a day program each morning. Dad had called me a few days after this placement, and I detected less anger and more fear in his voice, as I picked out the words, "pencil-pushing" and "school."

After getting the resident assistant on the line, I learned that the day program was geared towards seasonal, weather, and holiday orientation, and there were also crosswords and other aptitude activities for the residents to complete during their daily visits. The van left each morning promptly at 8:00 AM and returned at 3:00 PM. I quickly concluded that this was not going to fly with my father.

A few phone calls later, I had been able to convince the director that we would pay extra for an aide to stay back with Dad during the day, so he didn't have to participate in what he called the "r***** program."

This accommodation kept the peace for a while, but Dad had no love for the woman who ran this residence. He had many choice words for her when he would call me to complain, despite my reminders that she was there to take care of him.

While I may have been expecting reports of angry outbursts or using his walker as a weapon, I was not prepared for this May 1st call informing that Dad was in the wind. He had lifted the van keys from the ring by the door (who were they kidding, that was child's play for my dad!) and tried to make his way to Mendota Mental Health Institute.

Mendota was where Dad had already served several short stays, brought there against his will in the back of a squad car. Chris and I had worked tirelessly to find a residential home with the least restrictive environment, and he opted to try checking himself in to the most restrictive facility in the state? The only reason we could gather, was that at Mendota he was truly treated like a patient, whereas in the group homes he felt impaired and disabled.

The state troopers who were sent out to retrieve him told us later that he was doing all right on the interstate, he was maintaining his lane, and even signaled when they finally pulled him over. Once I learned that he was OK and that no one else had gotten hurt, I had to laugh a little and couldn't help thinking, "A for effort, Dad, way to go."

Needless to say, we moved him from that group home to yet another, where there was no more "school," and I hoped and prayed that we had finally found a good fit.

CHAPTER 70
Anything But That

Despite her ample waist, the nurse navigated the tiny examination room. She was a little out of breath, touchy, and motherly.

"My, aren't you just a sweetheart!" she cooed and gazed over my son's head at me with sympathetic eyes. She apologized with each poke.

Our little boy was stellar throughout the ordeal, as the nurse punctured him time and again, all over his back and arms, but by the end, he was starting to whimper.

"How many more, Mommy?" he asked when the nurse left the room with her metal tray of syringes and serum.

"No more, sweetie, we're done," I answered firmly.

We stopped after the environmental battery of tests, after pet dander, mold, and dust mites. I just didn't have the heart to go on to food. Two and a half hours and forty pin pricks later with no more answers than when we had first begun. After I called it quits, the nurse applied band-aids to the injection sites that were still bleeding, and then I helped him put his T-shirt back on.

"Any sticker you want, two stickers, okay? I'll be right back," promised the nurse.

The allergy specialist came in and straddled a squeaky leather stool. He rocked back on it and pored over my son's results, nothing of significance, a slight reaction to cats, a minor flare up to dust. The doctor smiled kindly at us both and suggested a special pillowcase, perhaps a duct cleaning for our home and stood up, signally the end of the conversation. I wondered if these were the standard suggestions given when the clipboard came back empty.

"Good day then," He said. He smiled again, shook our hands, and hastily exited.

As my husband Chris and I walked out to the parking lot I felt defeated. "Please, God, can't he be allergic to something?" I appealed to the universe. Lots of kids with allergies rub their noses, obsessively even. Allergies might make a child squirm and cough, I reasoned, and it would be rational and treatable, fixable, and controllable.

When the trouble started with our second son, we initially visited the pediatrician for a routine checkup. I thought the doctor might see something without me having to disclose my own genetic history. It was a fishing expedition at best, resulting in a co-pay to hear, "he's fine." Next, we met with his preschool teacher. She reassured us that children have slight nervous mannerisms all the time.

"It is perfectly natural and normal," she claimed, unaware that Huntington's disease lurked in the shadows, cackling at the uncertainty and paranoia of our days.

The allergist visit was the last stop on this route, this search for an alternative to HD. Before each of these appointments, I bargained with God, "anything but that."

It started with a cough of mysterious origin and no invitation, a little clearing of the throat, but to say that he did it three times a minute is no exaggeration. We tried to ignore it, but often found ourselves overcome. This morning I had lost it.

"Honey, could you just stop that coughing!"

I whipped around from the kitchen sink to see him jump and realized too late that I had shouted by the look on his face. I quickly put down the dish towel and shifted gears.

"What's wrong?" I asked, putting my hand on his cheek.

"There's just somethin' in my throat," he said, then shrugged and maneuvered from the breakfast table and out of the room.

It wasn't just the cough that plagued us. He rubbed his nose and squinted his eyes. He cocked his head sideways and rolled his left shoulder, rotating it like a pitcher warming up before a big game.

"Why do you move your shoulder like that?" I casually asked earlier this week.

"Because it just feels like I have to," he replied, and my heart sank.

"But why do you have to?" I pushed.

"I don't know," he answered stubbornly with the strained voice little boys use when holding back tears. I dropped it.

It's Turret's Syndrome, I thought, convincing myself that it must be. "Oh God, can it please be Turret's?" I pleaded for what I saw as the lesser of two evils. They have medication for that, and people can lead normal lives.

The pediatrician exam, the preschool conference and the allergist appointment were last ditch efforts of my denial that my son might have Juvenile Huntington's disease, a possibility I couldn't even bring myself to say out loud.

Juvenile Onset HD is rare, but real. According to the HDSA, this form of Huntington's is more known for seizures and rigidity than choreatic movement. I researched enough to know that the symptoms of early onset are different from typical adult cases. My son's symptoms didn't line up with these facts and yet, the connection between him, me, and my father seemed stronger than any factual barrier.

"Okay, buddy, let's go home. You were very brave today," I said.

I buckled him into his car seat, and Chris started the engine. As we drove, my memories travelled back to when I was the small child who wiggled.

My parents had talked, hushed but heated in their bedroom. Since the kitchen table was one paper wall away, I eavesdropped while eating my cereal.

"Leave her alone. I was twitchy when I was a kid, and my 'Old Man' always rode me about it," Dad argued.

"I'm just saying, it's a bad habit, and she needs to stop it," Mom returned. No answer from Dad.

"She looks ridiculous!" Mom pressed.

"Leave it be." Dad was defending me.

I drank the milk from the bottom of the bowl. It should have made me glow to have Dad in my corner, but a red flag waved. Somehow, I knew that I didn't want to be picked for his team. A dresser drawer slammed, ending the discussion.

I knew they were talking about me and the sliding glasses. Lately rather than push my glasses up when they slipped down, I just wrinkled my nose a little to the left and the right, a fine solution which repositioned them without having to pause anything my hands happened to be busy with. Great for bike riding, talking on the phone, latch-hooking, you name it, except that now I couldn't quit doing it.

I would order myself, "Okay, for the next five minutes, hold still."

I couldn't stop. Most of the time I didn't even know I was doing it, but when Mom gave me a look, I would jump and realize I'd been at it again.

"I think our courageous boy deserves a cheeseburger, what do you think, Mom?" Chris asked, looking over at me from the driver's seat.

I rose from my reverie as we turned into the McDonald's drive thru and saw a small smile from the rear-view mirror. We were twitchy kids, I acknowledged, Dad, and me, and now my son. Like the preschool teacher said, perfectly normal for a kid that age, but it was hard telling when my father's symptoms had started, and now his whole body was one constant movement, and I might be next.

A French fry waved over my shoulder from the back seat. I accepted the silent offering from his chubby hand but couldn't swallow it. There was too big of a lump in my throat.

Our boy was tired from the long afternoon at the clinic, so I changed him into his dinosaur pajamas and declared an early bedtime. That night held the darkest hours. I stood by his bed and listened as he breathed evenly, his mouth slightly open. He has beautiful long eyelashes, and they fluttered as he worked at slaying dragons in his dreams. I battled my own monster of fear.

"Please God, if someone must walk this path, let it be me. I will take it all, just don't let me have passed it on."

I was broken, bargaining, and begging. As I prayed, God drew close and met with me there, in the eye of the storm, as earthly forces whirled around me.

Spent of my tears, I touched his forehead gently and left the room. If I took the test for Huntington's disease, we could end this madness. It wouldn't change the future, but we could prepare for the days ahead. A negative result, and we were free. If positive, then our children would each have a 50% risk of inheriting HD, but we'd cross that bridge without shame and secrecy when we came to it.

Later that evening we sat on the couch and talked about testing. Chris held my hands and looked at me kindly but seriously.

"This has to stop. We can't keep chasing every angle, every 'what if' when the one unknown standing in front of us is the obvious question that needs to be answered."

I promised him that I would make some phone calls and find out the testing process, but I didn't want my grandmother to know anything about it. I didn't want her pressuring me or controlling my timetable. We agreed to leave it at that, and I am not proud of my procrastination at the expense of his patience.

As quietly as they arrived, our son's nervous habits

disappeared one day. Raising three young children, running a part-time business, and taking care of a home will cause you to often find yourself on autopilot. There were long stretches of time when I wouldn't give HD a second thought, until a phone call from Mom, or a clumsy accident from myself.

One night cleaning up after dinner I dropped a drinking glass, and it shattered across the floor. My eyes went out of focus as I traveled back to consequences from "The Book of Dad", and ahead to what I feared was a glimpse of my future. I clung to the kitchen counter inhaling deep gulps of air. Chris came up behind me and held me tight.

"Boys, it's okay, go play in your room," he said, then turning to me.

"Honey, it's alright. The baby is still in her highchair. No one's going to get hurt. Let me help sweep it up."

He sat me down at the table where I wiped back tears, took steady breaths, and comforted my baby girl who startled at the commotion. Quickly and quietly, Chris took care of the remaining fragments of glass, settled the kids in front of a video and came back to the table.

From the look in his eye, I knew what he was going to say.

"We have to know. Not because I'm going anywhere, but

I need to prepare myself, for what it's going to take to care for you."

He wasn't wrong. And yet, I'd held out for so long. I didn't want to know. I didn't want to admit that this could be what was going to happen to our family. I had worked so hard to make this family the complete opposite of the one I had grown up with. It was filled with sunlight, board games, and bedtime stories.

"You're right, I know," I conceded.

What choice did I have? I had to believe him. If we found out that I was positive, if I turned into my dad, would I blame him for running away, and sticking me in a home? I had to trust.

"Okay, I'll make the call," I said, and this time I meant it.

CHAPTER 71
An Advocate

Before Google was founded in 1998 and thereafter became a verb for searching in every household worldwide, finding phone numbers and resources took Yellow Pages or Directory Assistance. I found a toll-free number on the back of one of many HDSA pamphlets my grandmother had given me over the years. From there, my search took me to a social worker for the Wisconsin Chapter in the Milwaukee area, and I left her a shaky voice message indicating that I would like more information on HD testing resources in my area.

After ruminating on what I had recorded and almost regretting the call entirely, a few hours later, she returned my call. We spent the next 45 minutes on the phone discussing my grandmother's pedigree, the challenges that my family had been going through, and my father's recent diagnosis. Her voice was calm and reassuring, and she took intentional pauses and truly listened to me. I pictured her face and her eyes, and I imagined they were kind. We ended the call with a plan for me to make an appointment at a genetic testing clinic in Milwaukee. Once I had the appointment set, I should let her know, and she would meet us at a nearby coffee shop before we went in.

I didn't know how any of this worked. I asked her how we would pay for her services and her response was, "You don't, this is what we are here for."

In November of 2004, Chris and I entered the coffee shop, a swirl of warmth and the aroma of coffee beans contrasting with the damp, chilly air we had brought in with us. From across the room she looked up at us over her reading glasses and smiled. How had she recognized us? She was an expert in Huntington's disease, so did she detect symptoms in me already or were we merely the most apprehensive couple entering?

I had guessed correctly about her kind face and eyes, and she greeted us both sincerely and invited us to take a seat. Were we going to order anything? No, I couldn't possibly compound caffeine onto any shaking that my hands were already doing. She spoke, sharing wise advice about what to expect for the counseling session we were heading into. Chris took notes, and I struggled to remain present.

After we wrapped up our conversation, she gave us a few pamphlets, one about the genetic testing process and the other about a local support group. We thanked her and put on our coats.

"You don't have to face this alone," she said.

I know she meant it. Community and shared struggle help people through the darkest of trials, but I had never felt more alone.

CHAPTER 72
Solo Voyage

The sign at the clinic displayed services offered, "AIDS, Paternity, Huntington's." Everyone came seeking answers to their own private questions, and I avoided eye contact in the waiting area.

A woman with a clipboard called our first names, and my husband and I followed her to a conference room. The genetics counselor stepped in, closing the door behind her with a soft click and said, "Let's get started." With a gentle voice, she explained the testing process and the psychological impact of predicting your future. Chris actively listened and asked questions, while I struggled not to shut down.

We moved on to family history, and I pulled the pedigree chart from the manila envelope my grandmother had given me years ago. I shared printouts from her appointment at the Waisman Center as well as her hand-scrawled notes on those affected, those spared. I gave names and ages of our three children, anticipating judgment when the counselor recorded my daughter's birth date, two years after my father tested positive. No gavel banged.

"Noticing any symptoms?" She probed.

I admitted my struggle to focus, dropping things, and tripping, but withheld the anxiety attacks which gripped my chest and the depression that held me in bed after Chris left for work. She made notes and then closed my file, pausing.

"Do you want to proceed?" she asked carefully and held out an exit sign for a ramp that veered off called "backing out."

I glanced at Chris. "Whatever you want to do," messaged from his eyes.

"Yes," I answered determinedly, perhaps a little too quickly, and the phlebotomist entered in her crisp white lab coat.

"Follow me." She led me to a room much like those at my local clinic, where I had routinely sat in the plastic chair with the arm rest for sports physicals, my marriage license, and preventative care. Momentary discomfort, mere formality for almost certainly positive outcomes.

"You have nice veins," she remarked as she tied my arm off, and it pulsed. I tried to smile at her, but what do you say to that, "thank you?"

While she methodically labeled the empty vials and filled them one at a time, the realization hit me. My blood filled those containers, my name on those labels, my results alone. Imperceptibly things had changed. I had crossed over to a place where Chris couldn't follow, and I wouldn't wish so even for the excellent company it would offer.

In the lobby we paid with a credit card. Despite my husband's quality health insurance from the school district, these results needed to stay under the radar until we knew how to deal with them. I hastily signed the slip.

My future lay still warm in plastic holding tanks as we drove north toward home. A common band-aid marked the only sign that any of me had been removed, but the loss I felt was staggering.

Farewell to what the HD community calls the "tortured hope," for enduring the risk of being positive teams with the chance of being negative. One made the other bearable. In mere weeks, those two options would no longer live as roommates in my life, as one of them was about to be evicted.

CHAPTER 73
Waiting Period

The waiting period was six weeks. After the center processed the test results, we would schedule a return visit with a genetics counselor. My results would only be shared with me after undergoing an extensive counseling session to ensure I understood the ramifications of knowing my future. I agreed this was preferable to a depersonalized postcard in the mail, but it didn't make the waiting any easier.

Those weeks felt like years, but I did my best to stay busy and keep a routine. With caring for kids and running my consulting business, I was never short of things to do, but my mental capacity tapped out about three-quarters of the way through each day. By 4:00 PM, I was done.

I do not remember operating with my whole senses, it was more robotic, auto-pilot. Stirring some kind of dinner, putting plates out. Checking homework and breaking up arguments. I probably allowed too much TV time before running baths and tucking in.

Finally, the day came to head back to Milwaukee. The verdict was in. I couldn't eat the morning of, and I was trembling uncontrollably in the car. Even though Chris put his warm hand over the top of mine, it would not stop shaking.

We walked back into the clinic, and this time, I knew the drill. Check in at the counter, then wait in the uncomfortable plastic chairs for your name to be called, avoiding eye contact with all others in the lobby. It didn't take long for us to be called, and we sat down once again with the genetics counselor. I remembered her kind eyes, and she smiled at us both.

She held a manila envelope in her hand, and I couldn't take my eyes off it. She asked me how I was doing, and I said "fine," which is what you say when you're anything but fine. She explained in a few paragraphs the consequences of knowing your future and what it can do to you. She said sometimes not knowing is easier to deal with than facing a difficult truth, especially in the case of Huntington's, because although there are medications and treatments that have proven potential, there currently is no cure for this disease.

Did I understand? I nodded my head.

I kept trying to ascertain whether she was hinting at one result versus another in her comments, but she would have won at any poker table. There was no tell. Finally, after explaining everything that she had to say, half of which I barely listened to, she asked the question.

"Knowing all of this, are you still ready to find out your results?"

I looked over at Chris. His eyes were on me, encouraging, but waiting for my response. I knew he would respect my decision either way.

"Yes," I said.

She pulled a single sheet of paper out of the envelope. My heart was pounding, and time stood still. She set the paper down on the desk and looked it over, as if to remind herself of what the results were. Could there really have been so many that day? Or was it true, that the counselor really doesn't know your results either until she opens the envelope? After a pause, she looked up and smiled.

"I'm happy to say that your results are negative," she said.

I stared at her. Chris exhaled the breath he'd been holding and squeezed my hand tightly.

"So, there's no way I have it?" I asked once I found my voice. I was still skeptical.

"No, you are perfectly fine. Sometimes, if an individual has CAG repeats in the 30's, there can be a gray area, but you are a 17. That's about as low of a number as you could wish for," she explained.

She went on after that in greater detail, about my score and how it related to the CAG repeat continuum, but I had stopped listening. All around me was sunshine, beams of hope, an unbelievable lottery win. I had to tether myself down to the desk, back to reality, to my husband, the counselor, and the conversation we were having, for fear that I would float away. Not my former, disassociated float away to evade the scary, but on the sheer helium of a negative test result.

I started to pay attention again when she said, "So, let's talk about your symptoms, the reasons that brought you here in the first place, the stumbling, tripping, loss of concentration. You know they could be signs of something else going on with you, and I recommend that you visit your general practitioner, just to be thorough."

She gave her warm smile again and continued.

"But to be honest, why don't you take this good news and go home? Let it soak in for the next few weeks and see if those symptoms don't dissipate. Stress can contribute to mental health struggles. Physical issues can manifest as well, especially from the amount of stress that you have been carrying."

We wrapped up the paperwork, tucking my results back into the envelope along with a receipt for the services rendered, which we could now safely claim through our health insurance. Chris slipped it under his arm and held my hand as we exited the clinic. He opened my door for me and got me settled. I don't remember leaving the parking lot or heading down the road. I know we just kept looking at each other and smiling.

"Let's go get some lunch to celebrate," Chris suggested.

Suddenly, I was ravenous. "Yes, let's."

315

CHAPTER 74
Lunch on the Other Side

We stopped at a restaurant just outside of Menomonee Falls. I ordered something Mexican with chicken and rice. I sipped Diet Coke through my straw, and it was cold and fizzy. As we waited for our food we sat and looked at each other across the booth.

He couldn't stop smiling at me, and I would smile back, but trepidation which has held this tight of a grip for so long won't release that quickly. I feared it wasn't true, the results might be wrong, and that the clinic would call us later to admit there had been a grave and unfortunate mistake.

The place was packed for a Tuesday afternoon, people were gathered around the bar area watching sports on countless televisions mounted to the ceiling. Loud laughter filled the air, but it was as if I had been quilted, buffered from their noise and excitement. They were raucous and ignorant, but it wasn't their fault. How were they to know that today was any different from yesterday or from tomorrow? They were here for an early Happy Hour, and it didn't require much consideration.

My first thought was that I longed to be like these people, with their apparent lack of concern for the deep issues of life. I then realized I had both judged and stereotyped them, having no idea what paths these patrons might be walking when they left, perhaps this visit served as instant gratification or merely a band-aid for what waited at home. Maybe they were coping or denying something, and the truth was that I would not have traded with them and their seemingly carefree lot in life.

It was December 7th, 2004, and I found myself crouched at the bottom of a pit, gazing up at a speck of sun, and I would not have blocked that ray of promise for all the lighthearted pleasures of the world. It is the very marginality of such a fragment of light which offers immeasurably sweet reward, which cements you in gratitude. In addition to that glimpse of light, someone had thrown me a rope ladder, and now it was time for me to climb up and out.

Our server brought the food and warned of hot plates as she set them down. The rice smelled like Heaven and tasted like freedom. As we took our first bites, I remember the beginning of a conversation started by my husband.

"So, now what do you think we should plan?" he asked.

He continued, using more words than he often would

shed in a week. He dreamed out loud about going back for his master's degree, changing jobs, buying land, building a cottage, and taking a trip. I let him talk. So many times, I had squashed these thoughts, had often put my life, and in turn his, on hold, never daring to look too far into the future. In my defense, I often could handle no more than the next day. God had graciously given me each portion, doling it out as He saw fit. But today I cautiously allowed this exploration down a road that I had for so long deemed off limits. It was painful and exquisite at the same time. Eventually he paused to take a bite and asked me for my dreams, but I couldn't answer.

"Too soon," I said, and he nodded his understanding.

Lunch tastes different on the other side of disaster. If you chew slowly enough, you notice flavors that you swear were never there before. If you concentrate, new smells. As you swallow you can literally feel your body at work, that miraculous creation, with all its inner digestive workings. You take in nourishment and can sense its energy deposited in your limbs. You thank God for the food, ask Him to bless the strangers who prepared it, and then find yourself going even further, pleading with Him to care for all those who have less than you do on your plate.

As I savored salsa con queso I travelled outside of myself, and through the after-shift crowd and the roar of football on the big screen, I saw a world with God at work, and became lost in the mystery. I surfaced occasionally with a smile at this puzzle piece across from me and a nod to let him know I was listening. I marveled at this amazing counterpart given to me. My companion had notches of humanness that I somehow filled, as well as jutting edges of completeness that both strengthened and sustained me when I was at my weakest.

The adrenaline that had been summoned and gathered earlier in the day was now all dressed up with nowhere to go. I felt my body shaking as it tried to release the chemicals of fight or flight from within. Chris carried our take-out boxes and escorted me to the door.

It wasn't until we started the drive home that my muscles began to relax. Chris made a few cell calls, first to his sister who was watching our kids, the one family member we had confided in regarding our testing plans. Then he called a close friend with whom he had shared in confidence that I was finding out my results today. I listened in as he shared good news and felt myself drifting off into light sleep.

Where to go from here? "Too soon" was still my answer. I would think about all the ramifications and possibilities of a life spared later.

CHAPTER 75
First Call

My first call was to Grandma. I phoned the assisted living home, and the staff member put me on hold and went through the halls to bring the cordless receiver to her room.

"Hi Grandma, it's me," I said.

"Well, hello dear. It's so nice to hear from you."

"Grandma, I have news, and it's good news," I said quickly so she wouldn't start worrying.

"Oh?" she asked.

"Yes, you see, Grandma, I got tested for Huntington's disease, and I've been waiting for the results," I paused.

"I'm negative. I don't have it, and I wanted you to be the first to know."

There was a moment of silence on the other end of the line. I could hear her labored breathing, and I wasn't sure what she was going to say. Would she be resentful? I didn't think so, but I couldn't imagine anyone having HD and hearing someone else was negative, and what their external reaction would be, let alone their internal one.

I wanted to believe people would inherently wish the best for others, but I was new to my negative gene status and had never stood in gene-positive shoes. In that moment I had my first taste of what would become a steady diet of guilt.

Finally, her voice came, soft and choked with emotion.

"That's the best news I've ever heard. I'm so glad to hear that. So very, very glad."

"Thanks, Grandma. I wanted you to know."

"You've made me so happy," she said. "All I have ever wanted was for my children and grandchildren not to have this illness. Now I can be at peace and know that you and your family and all your future generations are safe."

It was the most gracious response I could have hoped for. My anger towards her that had built over the years dissipated as we spoke our farewells. I finally understood that all of her research and lectures were her desperate attempt to change fate and alter the course of the next generation. She likely held guilt of her own that she hadn't known what to do with.

We didn't talk much longer. I told her that I had a few other people I wanted to call, and I promised to talk to her again soon.

CHAPTER 76
Science vs. Feelings

I made a few other phone calls to family members and friends, but I don't remember much of the details. There was one I was dreading and delaying, but I knew I had to make the call to my sister. She picked up right away and asked me how I was doing. We hadn't talked in a while, and so we were catching up a bit before I finally worked up the nerve to switch topics.

"I tested for Huntington's disease. I just got the results back, and it's negative. I don't have it, and I wanted you to know."

It all came out in one pressured paragraph. And then silence, a stillness on her end even longer than when I was on with Grandma. So quiet to the point that I almost asked her if she was still on the line.

"Well, I guess I know what that means. I must have it then," she said.

"Wait, you know that's not true. You're a registered nurse. You know the genetics and the medical facts," I said, trying to counter her with logic.

Our entire lives my parents and other relatives had said I was the spitting image of my dad, while my sister resembled my mom. I had my dad's nose and was stockier, while her nose and thinner build came from Mom's side of the family.

Physical appearance has nothing to do with the genetic passing of Huntington's disease, but I battled that paranoia for years, thinking that because I looked like my dad, therefore I would inherit HD.

Another common misconception surrounds the odds of HD inheritance. It is easy to fall into the thought pattern that if one child of an affected parent is gene-negative, then the other child must be gene-positive, and if there are more than 2 children in a family, the odds would shake out 50/50 in some fashion.

Science tells us that each individual offspring has their own risk, their own coin flip, but I could relate to her immediate reaction. She felt that since I was negative, she must be positive.

"Yeah, I know it in my head. But that's not what my heart says," she said.

We spoke a little longer. I tried to reassure her of the scientific truths. That just because one of the coins flipped in my direction didn't mean the next coin would flip against her. But she was right, you can have all the genetic research and all of the science in front of you, and it doesn't change your heart or your feelings.

She talked about maybe getting tested sometime in the near future, but I could tell the motivation wasn't in her. We changed the subject and wound down, ending the call a few minutes later.

CHAPTER 77
God is Good

Since we seldom came to them, Chris's parents planned to travel to our house for Christmas that year. It was Chris's idea to wait a few weeks and share our good news of my gene-negative status in person.

We folded my test results in an envelope, told them we had a special gift for them, and handed it to his mother. Looking curious, she broke the seal and pulled out the single sheet of paper.

She was quiet as she read, and I could see her face change as the information took hold. Then she set the paper down on the kitchen counter and walked out of the room, overcome with emotion, and needing a minute to compose herself.

Chris's Dad picked up the results and read them for himself. Tears sprang to his eyes and a smile spread across his face as comprehension of this negative result sunk in. He pulled us both in for a big hug.

"God is good," he said, beaming, and then again, "God is so good."

The kids bounced around, hyped up on sugar and ready to open presents. Only our oldest really understood to the degree that Mom had taken a test for a disease, and she passed, she didn't have it.

Hugs all around, and it was a happy Christmas, but philosophical and theological questions kept nagging at me. Was God good because I was negative? If I had been positive, would He not be good? Why was He good to me and not to others like my grandma, her sisters, and my dad?

I don't pretend to know the answers to these questions. I did and do remain grateful.

CHAPTER 78
Survivor's Guilt 101

Don't call me a survivor. Survivors bring to mind images of people who, despite all the odds, have persevered, usually because of their own physical or mental, inner strength. Stories are told and media covers these types of stories. A climber, trapped in a mountain gorge, who pulled out a hunting knife and amputated his own limb to escape, then conjured a flare out of a bandana and some gun powder. This *MacGyver* was then rescued by helicopter and lived to tell his story to Barbara Walters on *20/20*.

I didn't feel like a survivor because I did nothing to earn this free pass. My genetic soup was simply stirred and out came a ladle of okay-ness. How did this make me better or more equipped than anyone else?

Psychologists and therapists call this emotion survivor's guilt, the incomprehensible sinking in that you have been spared, by whomever or whatever the powers that be, those gurus in the sky who determine whether you will live or die, by which method and when. You've been granted a stay, for how long, no one knows, but you better make the best of it. You shouldn't sit around and speculate, but you still can't help scratching your head, wondering "why me?" What have I got to contribute that ranks me higher on the list than those who were handed a positive test result?

Survivor's guilt is a response to an event in which someone else experienced loss or pain, but you did not. Although not considered an official psychiatric disorder, it is associated with post-traumatic stress. Survivor syndrome was first described in 1961 by William Niederland with respect to survivors of the Holocaust. Feelings about anything that I went through, when compared to someone having HD, let alone surviving the Holocaust, only produced additional, compounded guilt for feeling guilty in the first place.

For the past 30 years I had been traveling down one road, with one destination in the back of my conscience. It was a tragic location where I was heading to, but at least I had known the general direction I was going. Now, to U-Turn into the unknown was overwhelming, and I wondered, "What will I die of now? Cancer? A car-accident? How and when?" These questions didn't need answers, but they opened a door of uncertainty in my life, uncharted territory, whereas the original landscape had offered the minimal comfort of being known.

My at-risk status was intertwined with everything about me and contributed to the very fabric of my identity. Prior to testing, if I failed at something, I could say to myself, "Well, this must be an early symptom, surely I'm terminal with HD." Somehow that would make anything that happened explainable and acceptable.

Now, I was just like everyone else, and my mistakes, stumbles and careless maneuvers in this world couldn't be contributed to any genetic illness or destiny.

They were simply my fault.

CHAPTER 79
Giving Back

I began to look for ways to emerge from this slump. Since I was not affected, and therefore my family wouldn't be, maybe we could get involved and help the greater HD community?

My first step was to reconnect with the social worker who had helped with my predictive testing process, and she pointed me to the Wisconsin Chapter of the HDSA. We learned there was a hoop-a-thon fundraiser being held in Cedarburg, Wisconsin that year, and Chris and I packed up the kids and made a day of it.

I remember very little of my first encounter with the HD community. I was still processing my negative test result, contemplating next steps that had previously been on hold, and working through regrets of decisions that might have been hastily or impulsively made by a person convinced that their clock was ticking down more quickly than others.

We entered the double doors of a large gymnasium with bright lights and peppy music. People were milling around shooting hoops, raising money, and they all seemed to know each other and were already connected in some way. I felt like a stranger crashing their party and fought the urge to bail.

We approached a registration counter to turn in our fundraising forms and get name tags, and this is where I met Megan. I was immediately taken with her intriguing, icy blue eyes, which were complemented by a warm smile that welcomed us.

She introduced herself as the Regional Director of the HDSA and the person running this event. Then we met her mom, who was standing next to her. After introductions, Megan ended with, "and my dad has Huntington's Disease." She may as well have announced that we had been separated at birth, how strong those connecting words were, how they reached across the plastic table and wrapped me up tight.

We took our kids onto the highly waxed floor and found hoops to match their heights. Megan's daughter and mine instantly bonded the way little girls do, and they preferred dancing and playing Patty Cake on the basketball court to actually shooting the ball. Her beautiful daughter had the same bright blue eyes as her mother. Had she inherited anything else? I didn't know, and you didn't ask.

During a break, Megan's mom struck up a conversation

with me. She did not have the magnetic eyes of her daughter, but they were equally intense as she looked at me and asked hard questions. How was I dealing with my dad's health care needs? Did I have siblings at-risk? How was my mother coping? Rather than becoming defensive or guarded, I unpacked much of what I had recently been carrying, and we ended our interaction with a hug and her advice.

"You are a survivor. You fought the battle, and you won. Now, don't feel guilty about that, you just go on and live your life."

I left the fundraising event inspired and with determination. Megan was the first person I had ever met outside of my immediate family who was facing the same issues as me. If she could live at-risk and be this involved and brave, then I surely could live gene-negative in a more powerful way. I could advocate not only for my father and grandmother, but for the HD community at large.

The following year the HD Hoop-a-Thon was scheduled in Fond du Lac, but due to some snafu, the basketballs weren't available on the day of the event. Megan reached out to me, distraught and trying to hold a lot of details together, and asked, "Could we assist?"

"Yes, we can do that," I responded with confidence.

Chris and I went to the middle school where he taught, picked up a rack of basketballs, and transported them to the fundraiser just in time. At this second event I felt more comfortable and got to know a few other volunteers.

Megan and I remained in contact over e-mail, and I cherished those messages from someone who could truly relate. We talked about the anxiety, both of living at-risk and going through the testing process, hard pressed to say which was worse. We discussed remedies, mine was prayer, and hers was yoga. We shared stories about our fathers, and I was continually validated that I wasn't the only one.

Megan introduced me to other people in the HD community throughout the Fox Valley of Wisconsin. She was very connected like that, and much more outgoing than me. Through a mutual connection, I met the editor of the *HDSA WISCONSIN UPDATE* newsletter and wrote an article about my testing journey, When "Solo Voyage" went to print, Megan emailed me that same day.

"You have absolutely no idea how far you are going to take this," she wrote.

CHAPTER 80
Stage Fright

I set up my laptop and connected it to the projector, as lockers slammed, book bags thumped to the floor, and preteens yelled back and forth at one another in the hallway before lowering the volume and shuffling into the classroom to take their seats.

I gulped. I couldn't help thinking back to my freshman year of college when I spoke about HD to a room full of my peers. How their eyes looked back at me, some concerned, most disinterested, everyone uncomfortable. Would kids this age even understand or care?

I did not have a fear of public speaking. I had been presenting to audiences for years, through my professional career and also personally, at Christian Women's Club, and regularly for a large group of women who attended a weekly Bible study in our area. But these were middle schoolers, and I wasn't talking about Jesus. They were potentially going to eat me alive.

The teacher quieted the class down and began.

"I'd like you to meet the wife of Mr. Jones, my science teacher colleague, who many of you know. She is here to talk to you today as part of our genetics unit. She's going to talk about what it's like to live at risk and go through predictive testing for a genetic disease."

The students eyed me curiously.

"Mrs. Jones is going to talk about Huntington's disease, and I want you to pay close attention to what she has to say."

With that introduction and warning combo, I started.

"If you saw my father walking down the street in your neighborhood, you might cross to the other side. If you were with your friends, you might shove each other, giggle behind your hands, and point at him. You might think he was a drunk, staggering around, or that maybe he was high on drugs."

I paused and looked around at this audience, filled with kids who were between 12 and 13 years old. I could assume they had nothing more on their minds other than what was for lunch in the cafeteria that day or what video game they were going to play after school, or I could remember myself at that age, and the heavy fear I carried daily. Whether they were blissfully unaware or dealing with something at home, I needed to press on, and share my story.

"You would be wrong. My dad has Huntington's disease,

or HD for short. It is a fatal, degenerative, neurological disorder. Neurological means it affects your brain. Degenerative means it gets progressively worse. Fatal means it kills you."

The kids were quiet, rapt.

"HD effects approximately 40,000 people in the United States today, with another 200,000 who are living at risk. When I was your age, I lived at-risk. HD is autosomal dominant, which means if your parent has it, you have a 50% chance of getting it too."

I paused and brought up the slide displaying a Punnett square, which I knew the kids were studying. The teacher smiled from the back of the room as the students collectively groaned, because this was hard material. I also pulled a quarter from my pocket.

"Okay, let's break it down," I started, and we walked through how HD is passed, and I flipped the coin, having them predict heads or tails as we worked through the risk percentages. I could see in their eyes when they started to get it. This wasn't so bad.

I then demonstrated HD chorea and grimaces.

"People with Huntington's disease move their body uncontrollably, and they can't stop. They have trouble walking and with coordination, they have odd facial expressions, their eyebrows go up and down, and they might make noises with their throat or their breathing. They have problems swallowing and speaking. Because HD destroys your brain cells slowly, people with Huntington's may struggle making decisions and can show strange behavior. Because of all of these symptoms and its hereditary nature, having HD in your family has often been kept a secret, and families don't talk about it."

I moved on and shared the 1993 discovery of the HD gene on chromosome 4. I summarized, at what I hoped was a middle school level, how the DNA sequence of cytosine, adenine, and guanine (CAG) repeated over and over, the measuring of those repeats resulting in a predictive test for Huntington's.

I talked about how scared I was when I was their age, that I was going to get what my dad had, even though I wasn't really sure what it was. I then told them that eventually in 2004 I got the courage to get genetically tested. I explained that it was a personal choice, not everybody wants to know their future, and people need to respect that.

"My test was negative. I wouldn't get HD, and neither would my children."

Now they breathed a collective sigh of relief.

I closed with a wish that we could spread the word about HD to raise awareness and increase kindness.

"If you see someone walking or moving strangely out in your community, someone who looks different than you, please have compassion, understanding that there might be something more going on there."

Then I did the scariest thing. I opened it up for Q&A. The kids had prepared questions, and their hands shot up in the air. I don't know if there was extra credit for asking one or not, but I answered them all, surprised by how insightful they were.

The last girl I called on pointed at the pedigree chart which was the final slide of my presentation remaining on the screen and asked, "So, now that you are negative, if your sister is too, then is it, is HD, like, 'erased', from your family?"

I paused. That question had so many layers and answers under the surface. Would my sister test? And even if she did, would Huntington's ever be "erased" from my family? Never. But I knew what she meant.

"You are correct, no one could pass Huntington's disease on to anyone else in our family."

And then the bell rang.

CHAPTER 81
Popcorn

This is all about liability. This is all about covering their backsides. I came to this conclusion while nodding politely and listening to the caseworker's detailed discourse on the choking hazards of popcorn, on the risks of aspiration.

"Let me tell you about risk," I thought to myself, "I am intimately acquainted."

We sat in a dated conference room for the quarterly meeting, where guardians meet with social workers and clinical staff to determine the best way to care for the ward while maintaining a least-restrictive environment.

Everything about this room spelled "getting by," from the 1960's office chairs to the yellowed paint on the walls. The staff was weary, and their caseloads were heavy. My father was one of the "difficult" cases, a thick file of documentation on past behaviors and interventions. He'd been passed around, a hot potato that had landed in this unfortunate lady's lap.

It was quiet and everyone was looking at me. I realized that the caseworker had stopped talking, and that they were waiting for a response. As the silence grew, they shifted uncomfortably in their seats. I spoke gently yet forcefully, looking around the table, making eye contact with each caseworker, each health care provider.

"I'm going to have to disagree with your recommendation for a softened diet," I began.

The caseworker opened her mouth, as if to protest.

"You do realize he's terminal?" I asked them pointedly.

They nodded, offering a nonverbal retreat.

I continued, "The way I see it, our main goal at this stage should be keeping him comfortable. One of his favorite things is popcorn. Dad has always loved to snack on it, and it was an evening ritual in our house for as long as I can remember. Food is one of the only enjoyable things he has left, and I'm not taking away popcorn."

I paused. Despite my eloquent speech they didn't look completely convinced. "What do I have to sign to say that no one's going to get sued if he chokes?" I thought to myself. Was there a waiver for a terminal life's small pleasures, even if they might kill you sooner than expected?

We wrapped up. Papers were produced, documents were

signed, and the meeting concluded. We shook hands, and I found myself seated in the passenger side of our minivan with at best a fuzzy recollection of how I got there. My husband was buckling his seatbelt when the sobs started. He un-clicked his belt and wrapped his arms around me as waves wracked my body.

"Shhh," he quieted me. "It's okay, you made it through the meeting. You did great."

"It's not that," I said, wiping my eyes.

"Then what is it?" He asked. "You were a rock in there."

I looked up at him. "It hurts so much. It hurts so much more now."

"Now? What do you mean?" He asked.

"Now that I care."

He held me, and when I had come around enough, he let go, turned the engine, and we began the journey home. My own journey had started so long ago, and here I was, turning yet another corner. As badly as it wounded me to fight, to battle for popcorn for this man, I sensed a sweet washing over of God's pleasure, as if He were offering me a cool drink, a cold cloth for my head. As if He were saying, "I know it hurts to care, but that means you're healing."

I curled up in my seat and closed my eyes in emotional exhaustion, a *Velveteen Rabbit*, all beat up, frayed and worn, limbs hanging by a thread, holes in my side and fluff poking out. But real. Finally real.

CHAPTER 82
Plan Z

We had run out of options. The most recent group home where Dad resided had declared him a "difficult case," once again resulting in eviction. In desperation, I put in another phone call to the social worker who always picked up, the same woman from the HDSA who had been there to help me navigate predictive testing and gotten me more involved in the HD community.

Yes, she had a connection, one facility in mind where they might be willing and able to accommodate a special case. I made a phone call and set up a meeting with this residential care home in southeastern Wisconsin, which claimed to emphasize a flexible approach to healthcare.

"Flexible is definitely what we need," I told them when we met, and I didn't sugarcoat it.

I shared the difficulties we had encountered in many

homes before, Dad's frequent triggers which produced angry and sometimes violent behavior, his lack of filters and inhibitions. They seemed up for the challenge, so we signed the papers and initiated the transfer.

Chris and I traveled to the site to meet Dad's care team, and I wondered if this would be his last stop. Had we finally found a fit? As we pulled into the circular drive, the director walked out to greet us, with a bright smile and wide eyes that shone iridescent against his black skin. He had a slight frame and a melodic accent, and as I leaned in to catch his words, I could only imagine what my father would say about this mild-mannered man. My father was one rung on the ladder below Archie Bunker and let his opinions be known about colors or genders that were anything different than his own. How on earth was this going to work?

Despite my initial apprehension, Dad fit in here better than anywhere else, largely due to the staff's commitment in keeping to the age-old mantra our family held onto my entire childhood, "Don't upset your father."

The facility director, who would spend 18 years of his career with this agency, went to great lengths to educate his staff on how to meet the unique needs of those with Huntington's disease. My dad could not be rushed under any circumstances and needed ample time to communicate his needs. Much frustration and many outbursts could be preempted with a soft approach.

The staff understood that my dad had his days and nights reversed, and they were willing to accommodate. During his sleepless nights, Dad formed a relationship with a young man who worked the third shift so he could attend art school during the day. While the resident assistant spent the night shift sketching, Dad would sit at the kitchen table with a bowl of ice cream or a glass of milk and watch him draw.

While my dad could no longer control his hands, and they moved against his will, he could watch with his eyes and remember when he had been able to do drawings like this. They wouldn't say much, for once, my dad was quiet, but perhaps he took some comfort in living vicariously through the pencil and paper of that caregiver.

CHAPTER 83
Three-Volley Salute

The soldiers in dress uniform carefully folded an American flag 13 times into a tricorn shape and gently handed it to Grandma. She hugged it to her lap, hunched over in her wheelchair, and wrapped in a thick sweater.

Grandpa had donated his body to scientific research, so his military burial was delayed until the Spring after he passed away, and a chill remained in the air, as Chris and I stood with the kids at the cemetery grounds. My arms goose-bumped from the breeze, but even more so as Taps began to play. Nothing prepared me for what happened next.

An unfamiliar cream-colored minivan slowly approached our little group of grievers and pulled over. Out popped the director of Dad's residential home, and he levered open the sliding door and began helping my father out of the vehicle. To my amazement, Dad actually took his arm and stepped carefully onto the grass. My father wore dark navy sweatpants, a clean T-shirt, and his hair was combed back from his face. The clothes hung on his frame like a scarecrow's might, and his eyes looked milky and blank as he silently surveyed the scene in front of him.

My throat constricted with panic. I had sent over the details for the burial service, but I wagered that Dad would never agree to come, and yet here he was, swaying and fidgeting quietly at the back as the ceremony concluded. I jumped as the crack of the guns echoed in the air.

We brought the kids over to say hello to the grandfather they barely knew, and they awkwardly hugged him around his waist and then ran off to pick up the empty shell casings from the salute.

Never a more unlikely duo, I then watched Dad and the director walk together towards Grandma's wheelchair. Dad bent down and hugged Grandma around the shoulders. It was the first time they had seen each other since they had both been placed in care facilities.

Grandma and Dad held hands, exchanged final hugs, and possibly a few words between them. I worried that there would be a painful or embarrassing separation, that Dad would refuse to get back in the van and cause a scene, but when prompted, my father calmly accepted that it was time to go.

Years later when I asked about this particular road trip, the director simply smiled.

"When you sign up for this job, you are taking care of the entire individual, emotionally and physically," he said.

As I watched the van retreat, I marveled at the events of the day. I hoped they would take some country roads on the way back.

CHAPTER 84
Pro Bono House Call

Although the care home Dad was finally settled into went every mile to meet his needs, my father continued to push the limits of what most residential facilities were equipped and willing to put up with.

The staff would call when he was out of personal items and snacks, and while I could write checks and send supplies, I couldn't solve the biggest challenge, which was that my father refused to go to the doctor.

In a nursing home or long-term care environment, doctors come onsite and make regular rounds, seeing residents, providing treatment, and prescribing medication, but in this group home setting, the doctors insisted that the residents come to them.

My dad was currently on a long list of medications, including Lorazepam for mood and Morphine for pain, and his doctor rightfully refused to refill these prescriptions without first seeing him. Did my dad need Morphine for pain? It is hard to say, but there is significant research supporting that physical pain is very real for those suffering from Huntington's disease. A journal article by Sprenger, et al., 2021, published online in the National Library of Medicine, asserts that psychiatric issues in HD are often emphasized over physical pain, and therefore it is under-researched.

Those with HD may also have difficulty expressing their suffering, and therefore pain issues are ignored or overlooked. A series of abnormal pain events can occur and change as HD develops, including back, limb and abdominal pain, and a relationship between gastroesophageal inflammation and HD has also been explored. Here we thought that Dad was drinking Maalox by the bottle because of his abuse of ibuprofen!

In addition to pain, Dad was shrinking. Not since his intense diets during my childhood had I ever seen him this thin. According to Susan Sandler, M.S., R.D. in her article "Nutrition Intervention in Huntington's Disease," severe weight loss is a chronic symptom for Huntington's patients and can be aggravated by dysphagia (difficulty swallowing) which limits food intake, increased energy expenditure from chorea, and changes in psychological conditions causing appetite decline. An exaggerated number of calories is required to maintain weight, often as high as 3,500 to 5,000 a day.

How could we have a physician review his case when he refused to get in the van? The staff tried everything, from promises of rides in the country, to trips to get ice cream, but Dad wasn't going to be fooled. For a guy who had been obsessed with doctor's appointments and even high-jacked a group home van to get to Mendota, his heels were now dug in hard in the opposite direction.

"He's very territorial of the kitchen," the home director called and expressed this latest concern as well as a long list of others.

"Well, that's no surprise," I thought to myself, remembering childhood days of sneaking food so as not to poke the bear or make a mess that would result in a reckoning.

The director continued to elaborate on additional issues. Dad was become increasingly upset by loud noises, especially from the television and from another resident who routinely paced the perimeter of the home, shouting. He recently threw the remote control at the TV glass and cracked it. He refused to use his walker and was falling more often, then became frustrated when he needed assistance to get up.

But the biggest obstacle was that Dad needed his medication adjusted, it was vital that he saw the doctor, and he wouldn't go. If he got even a hint that a plan was underway, he shed his clothes and began throwing objects and breaking things or barricading himself in his room. I sensed we were at an impasse, but I promised the director that I would come up with something.

I then dialed a now familiar number. When I explained the situation, the HDSA social worker was quiet for a minute.

"I have an idea," she said.

"I'm all ears," I said.

An unconventional plan was hatched, and through a series of emails I came into contact with a since retired but well-known HD specialist. Would he be willing to make a house call? He agreed, and the date was set.

The morning of the meeting, Chris and I drove south to the group home, and I was a bundle of nerves. Would Dad refuse to see him? Or worse yet, would he become violent? We arrived and walked up to the home. It was a beautiful day, and an aide had brought Dad outside to enjoy the sunshine. The doctor pulled up just as we did and strolled casually over the lawn towards Dad, carrying a McDonald's sack.

"I shouldn't eat this stuff," he said sheepishly, and then he unceremoniously plopped down next to my father on the picnic table and offered him a French fry. Dad declined but remained docile as the renowned expert pulled out a stethoscope and listened to him breathe, then took a rubber mallet to his knees to check his reflexes. Finally, he patted him on the back and turned to us.

I sat in amazement as the doctor acknowledged and

validated both my dad's case and our situation. He shared that there was a newer medication called Tetrabenazine which could help with the chorea, but also had psychological side effects. Dad couldn't get on such a drug or participate in any clinical trials of others unless he actually visited a practicing doctor and cooperated with a treatment plan, but there were other things we could do. The doctor talked about caloric burn and recommended we start a daily protein drink. He also said that Dad could and should have all the ice cream he wanted.

We thanked him repeatedly, and after the doctor said goodbye, we stayed for a bit, Dad sitting quietly at the table, gripping the edge for support. I noticed the bruising over his forehead, his left eye, and running down his arm, the result of a recent fall. I made casual conversation and then circled around to it.

"You know, Dad, you should use your walker. It could help you not take so many tumbles."

He thought for a minute, then spoke so quietly, and muffled I could barely understand. I bent towards him to hear and asked him to repeat himself.

"When it gets to that."

"Dad, maybe it's 'to that'?"

He didn't answer, and I didn't press.

This pro bono visit didn't solve all of our problems, but I had never felt more heard, and I think Dad felt heard as well.

As I remember, the staff was finally able to get him to the clinic for prescription refills, and we took one win at a time.

CHAPTER 85
Interview with Grandma

After "Solo Voyage" was published in the HDSA Newsletter, I felt compelled to write more about Huntington's disease and my family's experience. There had been too much silence, shame, and secrecy. I called Grandma, the one person who was always willing to speak out, and she agreed to sit down and talk with me. I made the trip back to my hometown and headed to the assisted living home, but not before first grabbing her a snack.

It was late July, and nothing tastes better than beer-battered cheese curds from the County Fair. I picked up a package of the deep-fried cheese and then swung through the Dairy Queen for her favorite, a strawberry milkshake.

I had seen my share of group homes and care facilities, as Dad cycled through one placement after another, but my first impression of Grandma's residence was how nice it was, quiet and airy, with sunlight streaming through banks of windows in the dining area.

"Ah, so you're the author? The one writing the book?" The director sailed out of her office and greeted me, inviting me to take a seat at one of the empty tables. She smiled and said they would fetch my grandmother.

"She is so proud of you," she said with just a hint of "why don't we see you here more often?" in her voice.

A slight woman with a dish rag approached my table and began scrubbing it down. I quickly lifted my bag and the milkshake, and apologized for being in her way, thinking she was a nutritional aide with a job to do.

"Oh, you're good, that's just Alice. She gets a little anxious before dinnertime, so we help her find something to do with her hands," the director said.

I immediately forgave the earlier edge to this woman's voice and began unpacking my laptop, while a CNA went to get Grandma. It took a long time, but Grandma was never one to be hurried. When they wheeled her into the dining room, I couldn't help noticing how much she had declined. She was always heavier set, but now her skin hung on her shoulders, and she struggled to hold her chin up. But Grandma was all smiles when she saw me, and I gave her a gentle hug.

She smiled even wider when she saw the cone of battered cheese and milk shake. I shook a few tasty fried curds onto a paper plate to absorb the grease and placed the straw where she could reach it. I began my questions slowly, and her answers came even slower as she processed her responses and worked to say the words.

"I always knew, I always felt different," she said when I asked her if she worried about getting sick before actually testing gene-positive.

We talked about her sisters, how Luanne fell quickly with early and severe symptoms, Eilene next, and now her. We spoke about having children, and how hard it was for her to watch her own child begin to show symptoms.

Grandma told me that she had submitted our family history to the National Research Roster for Huntington's Disease, and we were just getting to the mystery visit, the day she took my sister and me for blood tests, when Grandma abruptly stopped talking.

Mid-sentence, Grandma choked, and I cursed my decision to bring the melted cheese. Her eyes grew wide, and I began to panic, but just as I was about to pound on her back and call for help, she brought up the bite, and I helped her spit it into a napkin. We held the straw, both of us with hands shaking for different reasons, while she took a sip of milkshake and recovered her breath.

I had so many more questions, but I could tell Grandma was tiring out, so I wrapped up the snacks and asked the staff to store them for later. Then I closed down the laptop, put away my notebook and gave her a hug goodbye. It was the last time I would see her alive.

CHAPTER 86
Team Hope 2009

The Hoop-a-Thon ran in Wisconsin for several years, and then the format switched to a national event called Team Hope, which is a 5K walk/run held in communities all over the United States, raising money for research and family support services.

Megan emailed me and asked if I could show her a park in Neenah where such an event could be held, and I knew just the one. I met her the following week with several volunteers, and we toured a park on the south side of the city, which had a pavilion, a playground, and a paved path for people in walkers and wheelchairs that ran adjacent to the Fox River. It was picturesque and she agreed it was a perfect location, and then she asked the burning question.

"Will you help?" she asked. "I need someone to run this event."

And I said yes.

No turning back now, I put on my operations hat and began to gather details. I first talked to the Parks and Recreation Department of our city, confirming a date for the event. Then I arranged to have the race route cordoned off on the day of, which was a Sunday and was going to cost extra. We looked at the budget, which was meager, and determined that we needed sponsors to pull this event off. I gathered a small team of volunteers, and we began to fundraise with local businesses.

Our kids made signs that read "We're Walking for our Grandpa," and they canvased the neighborhood raising pledges.

CHAPTER 87
First and Only Support Group Visit

y next stop was to the Huntington's Disease Support Group in Oshkosh, Wisconsin to promote the event, but I had no idea the effect that visiting this group would have on me.

I had never participated in an HD support group during the entire time that I was at-risk or going through testing, even though I had received information about it from the social worker in Milwaukee. It wasn't that I thought I didn't need it or wouldn't have benefited from attending, but my fear and decades of secrecy had always held me back. I contacted the individual who facilitated the group and learned when they would be meeting next.

On the day of the meeting, Chris and I drove to a hospital in Oshkosh and took the elevator to the third floor. We entered a small meeting room holding about 12 to 15 people, and I immediately detected that this was not just caregivers, but actual people with Huntington's disease.

I didn't know what to do with my eyes or my hands. I was frozen. I had never seen so many people in one room, writhing, grimacing, and shifting the same way my dad had for so many years. It was like looking at a ripple effect of him. I tried to slow my breathing. Chris touched my shoulder and pointed us to two empty seats, where we sat down.

The facilitator entered the room and smiled at everyone. Some people were obviously regular attenders, because she knew them by name, greeting them and asking about children and other family members. Her eyes then floated around the room and landed on Chris and me.

"I see we have two new attendees today," she said, politely and pleasantly.

"Um, I called you about the event?" I stammered.

"Oh yes," she said. "You are the ones running the walk-a-thon. Wonderful! We're going to give you a chance to talk about that in just a minute. But how about, first, anyone who's new introduces themselves. It's what we always do."

Great.

Chris went first, introduced himself and then said, "This is my wife."

I swallowed and went next, sharing my name and that my father had Huntington's disease, and my grandmother did as well, and my great aunts and another cousin that I knew of. I was here to share about an event that was being started in the Fox Valley to raise funds for research and community support.

I couldn't help thinking that these people must be wondering why I hadn't shown up until now. Why had it taken a negative test result to get involved? Why had it taken 5 years?

"Why don't you go ahead and tell us about the event now," the facilitator suggested.

I stood up and passed out the materials, telling the group about the 5K walk/run that would take place in Neenah in August. If they had any questions they could contact me, but I hoped they could attend and spread the word as well. It was not my best work. I felt like everyone was looking at me, as if to say, "Well you're fine. What are you doing here?"

I quickly sat back down, and then the topic for the session was introduced by the facilitator. She passed out more informational material, and some people participated in her questions and discussion, but I don't remember what we talked about.

I averted my eyes to the chorea that surrounded me, but the attendees simply acknowledged it. There were two sisters of a brother who had HD, and they shared honestly about their situation, not only his decline, but their own struggles in caregiving and navigating the healthcare system. He sat between them, with his eyes downcast, and it felt somewhat disrespectful. Was he aware that they were talking about him? Or was he floating away? Had HD taken so much of him already that he no longer sensed his loss of dignity? Or was being here, present in this group, the ultimate preservation of dignity?

I had never witnessed such an openness about Huntington's before and waffled between admiration for their authenticity and wanting to crawl out of my skin.

I was anxious to leave when it was over, and as we drove home, Chris could tell I was not okay.

"That was really hard for you in there, wasn't it?" He asked.

I shrugged and tried to downplay it, but he always sees through me. I sat quietly but then finally spoke.

"Yeah, that basically sucked, and I don't know if I can do this. I don't know if I can chair this event. I feel unqualified and like I don't deserve to be here. I still feel like I don't deserve to be negative." The old Survivor's Guilt had reared its ugly head, like a monster which feeds on itself.

"Lori, if the negative people don't help the positive people, then who will?" he asked.

I knew he was right, and I knew we would run this event. Despite my fears and the churning in my stomach, we were going to make it happen.

CHAPTER 88
Race Day

The morning of the first Team Hope, Fox Valley event promised sunshine and a beautiful almost autumn day. We set up a stage and a banner and wrote all the team names on a whiteboard behind it. The T-shirts were folded and waiting at the registration table, prizes were set out in the shelter house, and I paced around a nervous wreck. What if no one showed? What if we went to all this effort and raised no money?

And then people started coming.

Cars pulled up, medical vans with people in wheelchairs and walkers, their family members helping them slowly approach the pavilion. Someone turned on the music, and it began to feel like a party. People were everywhere, signing up at the registration table, writing their donation checks, putting on T-shirts, and taking group photos. Race bibs were pinned to the backs of those running, and some athletes were already stretching, while the casual walkers were drinking coffee and eating donuts. It was a brilliant mix of family members, caregivers, and affected.

I stood speechless, once again surrounded by people like I had only ever seen in my family, and I fully realized that we were not alone. I saw Great Aunt Luanne depicted in a young woman's arms, flailing, and circling as if she were dancing, her fingers pressed to points like she was playing castanets. I saw my grandmother's classic sway, back and forth, as an older man appeared to rock a baby. Another woman displayed Great Aunt Eilene's smile, her too wide grimace and curious eyebrow raise. Then I choked up when I saw a younger man, shuffling along in a track suit, completing my dad's signature move, swiping his hair back from his forehead, subconsciously compensating for his chorea.

I started to relax and interact with a few people, and as I walked over to the food table to check on our business sponsors who had delivered the snacks and meals, I saw a group I recognized coming up the path. Here came my extended family from the farm. Great Aunt May, who had experienced some other than HD health problems and aged since I last saw her, wore dark sunglasses, and made her way carefully on the arm of her oldest son. She had brought her sons and her daughter Bea with her, and Bea had brought her oldest son as well. They were here. I couldn't believe it.

Great Aunt May hugged me and said hello.

"We brought a donation," she said quietly, clutching an envelope, bulging with cash, and taped shut. "I'd like to make sure it gets into good hands."

"Come with me," I told her, and we went to the registration table so that she could hand over what appeared to be a sizable amount of money.

The race was run, prizes awarded, donations tallied. Our small team of volunteers cleaned up as the last participants hugged goodbyes and made their way to their vehicles.

This day marked many firsts. The first Team Hope event held in the Fox Valley. The first time I saw my family openly identifying with and united against Huntington's disease. It was the first time I had felt part of a greater community, a shared struggle, and although I was bone-tired, it was the first time I can remember not feeling angry or scared.

CHAPTER 89
Organ Donor

Grandma passed away in July of 2012, and I felt guilty for not having been back to my hometown to see her before then, and that the news had passed from one family member to another until it came my way.

Grandma had chosen not to donate any of her organs for scientific research. As progressive as she had been, educating herself on the latest developments and subscribing to the HDSA newsletters, towards the end of her fight, I remember her saying, "This disease has taken so much of me. I'm not giving any more."

Perhaps it was her strong Catholic background that contributed to her refusal, or maybe she was simply resentful and angry. I remember Grandpa being annoyed and frustrated that she wouldn't complete the donor paperwork when he did, but he didn't fight her.

I needed to tell Dad that his mother died and considered

the best way to do so. Our in-person visits with him had dwindled to the on-site quarterly reviews that we held with the county caseworkers, and I dreaded them. No amount of preparation or self-talk made it easier to enter the group home. I have no doubt the staff was doing their best to care for the residents and their specific and challenging needs, but I was always met with chaos.

Usually the TV was on a steady stream and an aroma of left-over lunch lingered in the kitchen, where we would gather around a sticky Formica table and sign off on forms. During our meeting, inevitably someone was screaming or banging their belongings or body parts against a surface, expressing discontentment. Despite the gallons of disinfectant they must have gone through, there was always an underlying odor of urine and refusal to bathe.

I felt bad for not seeing Dad more often, but life was busy with three kids, and we had to arrange their schedules and take time off work to make a day trip. In truth, the kids were scared to go, and I didn't want to make them. His appearance and behaviors frightened them. In truth, I was also scared to go. His appearance and behaviors still frightened me.

Even after testing gene-negative and knowing that I wasn't looking at my future on fast forward, seeing Dad still resurrected stress and trauma, and I regressed back to my childhood self every time. On our return trips home, I would curl up and sleep, and for days after each visit, I would be out of sorts.

In the past Dad would sometimes come out and sit down with us during our meetings, but lately I'd have to go into his room to find him. After he recognized me, he would hold on tightly to my arm and get uncomfortably close. Desperate to communicate, he would force out words or use his hands to gesture, and he became angry if I couldn't understand. He often followed us out, and it was difficult to leave.

How would I tell him? How would he handle this tragic news, a man who became distraught and combative over empty ice cream cartons?

But I couldn't keep it from him, so we made the trip, and I mentally prepared for it over the miles we drove. When we entered through the front door, an aide greeted us pleasantly.

"Your dad is lying down, but I told him you were coming, so go on in."

I peeked into his room and saw him dozing with a thin blanket pulled up to his chin and covering his wasted body. He was almost skeletal and unresponsive when I said his name. I sat down next to his bedside, shaking his shoulder gently to wake him. He opened his eyes slowly and gazed at me. There is no instruction manual for how to do this, so I launched in.

"Dad, I came to tell you that your mom, Grandma, died this past week. She was getting sicker, but now she's not suffering anymore. I know how much she loved you and how much you loved her."

I paused and let him take it in. His cloudy eyes studied me as he processed the information, and then he exhaled heavily, nodded his head, and closed them again. He took my hand and held it tightly. We stayed a few minutes longer, until I could tell he had returned to sleep, and I slipped my hand from his grasp. As we got back in the car, it was with a mix of relief that the visit had gone without conflict and a profound sadness that it had been that easy.

On the way home Chris and I talked about organ donation. My grandmother's passing and my father's steady decline had once again stirred the consideration of a donation for research. I had learned about organizations that did this through the HDSA, but had kept it on the backburner, thinking we had plenty of time.

The next week I followed up with the Harvard Brain Tissue Resource Center (HBTRC.) The HBTRC was established at McLean Hospital in 1978, known as the Brain Bank, and acting as a centralized resource for the collection and distribution of specimens for research. I spoke with their staff at length about the program and what a donation would mean for scientific study and a cure, and they assured me that the process would be handled efficiently and at no cost.

As my father's guardian, I could sign off on a brain tissue donation, but it was with mixed feelings. I remembered how he felt about Grandma's research, and how the blood samples we gave as children were done secretly so as not to upset him. I could only hope that He would have come around, knowing this could help future generations. With so many obstacles against him, this was one gift that he could give, a legacy he could leave, so I made the decision to proceed and signed the forms.

CHAPTER 90
Comfort Measures

The group home director called and said it wasn't good news, but seriously any time he called, was it ever good news?

"Your father has taken a turn," he said quietly. "It's looking like it might be getting close to the end."

"What does that mean?" I asked.

I knew we'd been headed for this day, but now that it was here, I felt flustered and unprepared.

"I recommend you consider placing him in Hospice care," he said and explained the details in transporting Dad to a place where people could keep him comfortable.

I agreed, and we worked out the logistics of the transfer. For once, we didn't have to strategize about how to sweet talk him into the van or get him into clothes and out the door. Dad had declined too much to fight, and mixed with my gratefulness was sadness. I couldn't picture my dad without his feist.

Knowing time was limited, we arranged a trip for the whole family to the Hospice facility in Whitewater, Wisconsin. As I entered the building, I couldn't help noticing it was aged and broken down, it smelled musty, and the carpets were stained. The workers looked tired, career smokers with home perms, but they were unfathomably kind, and I immediately felt small for judging them and this place. They gently prepared us for what we would see before we went into the room.

Mom was going in first. She hadn't seen him in a long time, so I was worried how she would handle his emaciated state. Would he be awake enough to communicate with her? And if he was, how was that going to go? She spent what felt like quite a while in there with him while we waited in the narrow hallway. When she came back out her eyes weren't dry, but she looked relieved, resolved, and at peace. Yes, she nodded, they had been able to say their goodbyes.

It was my turn to go in, and I thought I was prepared, but wasn't. He was a skeleton with skin. I was rooted to the entrance, unable to move. How could he possibly have gotten this frail in the last month? He took in ragged breaths with his mouth half open. He hadn't been wearing his dentures, and it had only taken a short time for his gums to collapse in on themselves like an expired carved pumpkin. His eyes were rheumy slits.

I forced myself to sit down beside him and picked up his

hand, which was paper thin.

"Dad, it's me. I'm here."

No response. They had told me, "talk to him like he can hear you," and so I did. I told him that everyone was here to see him, that we loved him and that he should keep resting and not feel like he had to talk. After a while I got up and left so that the kids could come in with Chris, but first I pulled my husband aside.

"Are you sure about this? Are we sure we want to do this to them? I don't know if they're old enough to handle it," I said my voice tight with emotion and panic.

"When are they gonna be old enough to handle it?" he asked. "They need to see him now, or they'll never see him again."

"But is this how we want them to remember him?" I asked.

We looked at each other seriously for just a couple minutes, and then we silently nodded in unison. They needed to see him like this, even if it was hard. This was their grandpa, and this was his fight.

Chris filed the kids in, and they stood in a row and told Grandpa they loved him. It was brief, and they beat a hasty retreat out of there. I still don't know if it was the best decision.

"How much time do you think he has?" I asked the Hospice worker as we prepared to go.

"Well, one never knows how long someone might hold on," she answered ambiguously.

I hated the uncertainty of it, and yet a part of me clung to the uncertainty of it. When I pressed her further, she shared that, while she could not predict anyone's passing, she wouldn't recommend letting more than a day or two go by before coming back if we wanted to see him alive again.

We drove back home, the kids falling asleep in the back seat, everyone exhausted from the emotion of it. Chris and I talked quietly about the logistics, when and how we would get back down to sit with him, and about the many arrangements to make after he passed. I didn't ask but sensed my mom was done, and she wouldn't be back.

CHAPTER 91
Fuzzy Angels

When I was a young girl, we went to church in an old brick building downtown. Squeaky hardwood floors, pews shined and slippery with furniture wax, where my feet swung because they couldn't reach the floor. While the organist played, I'd look up at the cathedral ceilings and the stained-glass windows which seemed to reach the sky, and I would anticipate the bell that the usher pulled with a rope, ringing us to attention.

We went to the old brick church back when Dad sometimes came more often than Christmas, and in my earliest memories there, church was led by an angel.

From the pew I sat in, always the third row from the front on the right, beamed a fuzzy, luminous, white, flowing creature. His shiny silver face radiated golden beams of light and from it, a soothing voice, deep baritone, and hypnotic, which rose and fell with his points and passion. I knew when he wound up that he was winding down, hands in the air, waving the benediction.

"May the Lord bless you and keep you, The Lord make his face to shine upon you and be gracious to you. The Lord lift up the light of his countenance upon you and give you his peace; and the blessing of God almighty, the Father, the Son, and the Holy Spirit, be among you and remain with you always. Amen."

It turned out that in the third grade, what I really needed was glasses. When it came to my turn in the receiving line, Pastor D. materialized into human form, wings tucked away, but his eyes twinkled behind gold rimmed glasses, an ever-present smile on his face and a warm grip as he held my small hand in both of his giant ones.

"How are you today, young lady?" he asked. He would bend over, low to the ground and look square in my face, seeking a real answer.

Dad had liked Pastor D. I remembered their warm handshake on Christmas Eve many years ago. Mom said that they used to hang out together, sometimes go to Madison, and even went sailing.

Was it too much to think that Pastor D. might still be in the business of angel-ing? If there was anyone who knew my dad enough to hold a memorial service, it would be him. I had to find him, but I had no idea how.

Thankfully, my mother is active on Facebook, and she

had a connection of a connection, a long story that turned into a way that I might be able to contact him. It was slim but worth a try, and never a stranger message had I composed to anyone before.

What would I say? "Hi Pastor, remember me, I was a nine-year-old little girl with nearsightedness and a lot of family trouble? Do you happen to remember my father?"

I crafted a message to him asking if he remembered my dad. I told him that Dad was currently in Hospice in southern Wisconsin, and that it didn't look like there was much time. I hit send.

The response came almost immediately, and he gave me his phone number, asking me to call him. I sat in my kitchen and dialed the numbers with trembling fingers. His deep voice, just as I remembered it, picked up on the first ring. Yes, he remembered.

We spoke for a while, and I asked him if he'd be willing to do a memorial service, as my father didn't have much time. He said he would be honored and that he was still in the area and would try to get over to the Hospice facility to see Dad if he could yet this week. This was more than I expected or even hoped for.

Pastor D. shared how close he was with my dad and that he was a support system to him in his hour of need. I wasn't sure what that meant, but we ended the call, and I felt real hope for the first time in days.

Later that week, the message came through that Pastor D. had been able to stop by the Hospice center, and yes, he did think that my dad recognized him. I expressed how grateful I was to him for that visit and told him I would stay in touch as to the timeline.

CHAPTER 92
Memories Pressed

The Hospice workers gave us free reign in the room and told us to relax and sit with Dad like we were hanging out during any other normal family gathering. Little did they know that a normal family gathering hadn't ever happened in all of my memories.

Dad had never just hung out and relaxed, his limbs and his mind were never still, and so it was ironic that the last hours I spent with him were his most peaceful and mine.

Chris and I loaded a Presley soundtrack on Pandora and got to work, using my laptop to create the slide show that would run during the service. We cracked open photo albums, as Elvis sang about memories, pressed in these pages, and also in my mind.

We reminisced and held photos up to Dad, talking like he was looking right along with us. Sifting through mementos, I found the small yellow cardboard square, with a pressed dandelion and an inscription on the back. Dad's gift when I was four years old had traveled with me in a keepsake box to college, multiple apartments, and into my married life. Forty years later, and I still kept it close. It sits on my desk today.

As we wound down, I knew that it was getting late, and I was going to have to go. Chris planned to stay, and I was driving home to see to the kids. Chris would tell me later that he knew he needed to be the one to be with Dad when he passed away. It was the one thing he knew he could do for me that he didn't think I could do on my own.

I don't know, I might have been able to do it on my own. I've done so many things on my own before, but sometimes you have to accept what people want to give you, not only for you, but also for them.

CHAPTER 93
Brain on Ice, August 2013

The upstairs parents' lounge of our community gymnastics center had no air conditioning, but two industrial fans were blowing the damp air around the room, which smelled of chalk dust, sweat, and rubber gymnastic mats. I tried to focus on my laptop and the work at hand, for which I was so incredibly behind, and every so often peaked down from the observation deck to the lower floor, where my daughter was running through her tumbling routine. She landed a round off, looked up at me and waved. I gave her a thumbs up and a smile.

The call came in. My cell phone volume was maxed, so as not to miss any calls from Chris, and it gave a jarring ringtone that made me jump as well as other parents who were waiting in the room and watching their own children.

"It won't be long now," he said. "I'll call you back as soon as I know."

We ended the call, and I sat in both shocked and yet unsurprised silence. All around me parents made small talk about their child's progress on the balance beam or what their family was doing for the upcoming Labor Day weekend. Mothers consoled whiny younger siblings with Goldfish crackers and promises of leaving in five more minutes.

I knew it was coming, but now that it was here, the finality sunk in. "I should be there" is all I could think, even though we had arranged that I would come home and get the kids back on their normal routine, while Chris stayed and kept me updated. I had reluctantly agreed to that plan, knowing the kids needed Mom and feeling a bit relieved to no longer watch the clock hands rotate in that Hospice room. Dad's cousin Bea was there too, taking turns sitting with him, and Chris said she was now reading Psalms and reciting the Lord's Prayer.

The second call came in, as loud as the first.

"He just passed away," Chris said these words quietly, I had to press the phone to my ear to hear him above the lobby noise.

He continued, "I'm going to wait here. Bea went home, but I'm waiting for the donor transport to come. It seems there's a delay, the courier vehicle is running behind, and they've asked me to pack him in ice."

"What?" I asked, incredulous, "What are you talking

about?"

"We need to keep the brain cold. We've got ice bags wrapped around his head, but they keep slipping, so I will hold them there until the transport comes."

When we initially arranged the tissue donation, we had been given a number and instructed to call immediately after he died to arrange pick up. When he called, Chris received specific instructions to keep the brain cold until the transport arrived, one bag of ice on the side of each temple and one laid across his forehead. Chris told me that the ice began to melt, small rivulets of water dripping down his father-in-law's face.

Chris's immediate thought was "I should wipe that," followed by, "That's silly, he isn't here to mind." Chris took a towel and wiped the water anyway, as it seemed like the right thing to do. After over an hour of sitting with my dad on ice, the team arrived.

I was stunned and had no words. What do you say when your partner in life is willing to sit in Hospice care holding your father's head in bags of ice until the Mortuary Transporter arrives?

We exchanged goodbyes, "I love you's," and I clicked off. I needed to remember the tasks at hand. I would collect my daughter from gymnastics, assure her well done, regardless of how many times she stumbled, or didn't stick the landing. I would tell her no, no French fries tonight, we have food at home.

I needed to get home and make dinner for the boys. They were old enough, it's not like they couldn't cook a pizza, but even adolescents feel the strain of a broken routine, and ours had been in shattered pieces for the past two months. I mostly needed to make sure they weren't fighting.

The house was a mess from our days away. Everyone needed baths, homework checks and tuck in routines.

"Then and only then can you cry," I told myself.

But by the time all the to-do items were ticked off the list, the children were in bed, and I sat on the couch, I couldn't find any tears.

I waited for the call from Chris to tell me the pick-up was done, nodding off despite my best intentions.

The phone rang, stirring me from sleep.

"It's done," Chris said. "I'm on my way home."

"Please drive safe," I said. I looked at the clock and saw it was close to three in the morning.

"I will. I picked up a Mountain Dew for the road," he said.

We hung up, and I climbed into bed. Hours later, I felt his arm wrap around my waist, holding me tightly.

CHAPTER 94
Ghostbusters

Events after happened quickly. I had several phone calls and many preparations to make, my first task being to call Pastor D. and arrange a memorial service. Yes, he did have the date we had been contemplating free, but he had an afternoon engagement, so he'd be coming in hot. Could we hold the service until about 6:00 PM? He asked.

Of course, I could. I would hold as long as necessary for that man to get there.

The night before the funeral, our family gathered with my mom and my sister and her husband and all of her children, who had traveled from Michigan, and even Chris's parents came as well. We drove out to Cadiz Springs, had a meal in the shelter house, and then and in honor of Dad, we took a lap around the lake. My gangly adolescent children humored their mother, swatting mosquitos and trekking around this relic of my past, my oldest watching me intently in a curious and protective manner.

The next day was filled with preparations for the service. Chris and I went to the grocery store, stocking up on Junior Mints, Hostess Twinkies and HoHos, all the treats that Dad loved best. We set out the snacks, decorated the room at church with photos, and started the slide show running, with the Elvis hymns playing in the background.

People began filtering in, and I was surprised and humbled by each connection from both my past and present. The special family from my high school years arrived, who had taken me in and carted me everywhere, including to camp each summer. Then the director of Dad's most recent group home, the one who had driven him to Grandpa's burial and navigated doctor visits and end-stage logistics, slipped in quietly and took a seat.

As the clock drew closer to when the service was supposed to start, I kept reminding myself that he said he would come, and he did. Pastor D. rolled in about ten minutes after, having ridden his motorcycle, his hair was swept back as he pulled on his ministerial garb. He looked older but exactly as I remembered him, minus the blurring fuzz of near-sightedness, sporting a long robe and hemp rope tassels around his neck.

The attendees quieted in their seats as he took the stage and got right to business assuring us, this little band of people who had walked the path of Huntington's disease with my dad, that he was okay and in a better place. I wasn't ready to believe that. My dad had told me on more than one occasion what exactly I could do with my ideas of faith, church, or any of that other BS, and yet here was Pastor D. telling us about midnight calls when Dad couldn't sleep.

"It was the middle of the night when the phone rang," he began.

"I picked up, but the caller wouldn't speak. I tried asking who it was and how could I help, but all I heard was labored breathing."

Pastor D. shared that these calls came regularly for several nights in a row, and he continued to pick up and speak to the silent caller. Something told him to stay on the line.

"I said that I was here for them, and I prayed for them. Then it would be silent and eventually the caller would click off. After about a month of this, the caller finally spoke and identified himself as the man whose life we celebrate today."

So began a routine, when the night demons were chasing my dad, he picked up the phone and called his pastor and friend. During those midnight calls Dad confessed his fears, fears of trying to raise a family, of having a wife and two beautiful girls that he loved so much, but "The Shakes" were coming. He was getting "The Shakes," he could feel it.

Pastor D. couldn't promise "The Shakes" away, couldn't reassure that his symptoms wouldn't get worse, and that things wouldn't end badly, but what he could promise him was the peace of God to make it through.

On those middle of the night calls they spoke of love, and how God's love would give him the peace and strength that he needed to live these hard days. At the end of Pastor D.'s message, he once again wound up those arms for the benediction, the sleeves of his robes billowing with the gesture.

"So, I ask you," he said, looking intently at the people gathered.

"I'm going to ask you. In the middle of the night, when you are afraid of the demons that are chasing you, when all of your fears coming closing and crashing in on you, who are you going to call?"

My middle guy sat on one side of me and my oldest son on the other, and they punched me softly in the side and grinned. All smiles they whispered, "Ghostbusters!" after the iconic movie tagline, and the three of us started to shake with laughter, silent laughter (this was a funeral for crying out loud!)

I thought to myself, "Dad wouldn't have wanted it any other way, us cutting up in church."

CHAPTER 95
Team Hope, September 2013

We hadn't really planned ahead for this, and it felt strange, like crashing a wedding. When we arrived at Team Hope, Fox Valley, we saw what we knew to be hours of preparation and planning for which we hadn't been involved in or contributed to. We hadn't even attended the past few years.

We approached the registration table with a check. A volunteer I didn't know took our names and contribution, her eyes widening a bit at the figure, which was half of the memorial fund from Dad's funeral. The other half was going to place a bench at Cadiz Springs, along the trail that he so loved to hike.

Chris and I put on our T-shirts and waited for the send-off to make our 5K laps around the park. I gazed around, and it still amazed me, watching people mingling, supporting the cause, talking openly about having HD. Whole communities arriving to support their friends and family.

And then I thought I saw my long-time friend Lauren. What would she be doing here? When our eyes met, she ran over to me.

"Oh my gosh, you're here!" she pulled me into one of her fierce hugs.

She shared that she was there for a man in their neighborhood, a husband and father who had just been diagnosed with Huntington's disease. Their whole cul-de-sac had come out, rallying behind their neighbor and friend.

"How is your dad?" she asked.

"Probably better now," I said. "He passed away last month."

She hugged me again, and I began to tear up. We caught up a bit more, and then she left to go find her group, as I wiped my eyes and tried to compose myself. Chris stood quietly by, recognizing this was the first time I had cried since my father died.

"It's okay to be emotional about this. It's okay to grieve," he finally said.

"I know," I said, using the tail of my event T-shirt as a tissue and feeling relieved when the airhorn sounded, signaling the crowd to take off.

After putting in our miles, we stayed a bit and picked up some submarine sandwiches and water bottles. Surveying the tables for a place to sit, I saw an older but still familiar face. Could it be? We made our way to her table.

"You likely won't remember me," I started. "You see so many people and so many families, but I wanted you to know that you were a huge help to me and my family during our time of need."

I told the social worker who I was, reminded her of my predictive testing in Milwaukee, and shared that my dad just passed away last month.

"He wouldn't have had the care that he got in the last few years without your help and your network of connections," I said, thanking her.

I felt like a student, running into a former teacher, and telling them what an impact they have had on their life. She smiled humbly and told me that she had since retired from the HDSA, but still came to events. She said she couldn't completely check out.

We left the fundraiser shortly after talking with her, feeling spent and yet full. Would I be checking out? Was this the end of my journey with Huntington's? Had I assuaged my Survivor's Guilt and filled my philanthropic cup? I wasn't sure, but this had been a good day, and I committed to remain in the present and not think too far ahead.

CHAPTER 96
Christmas Day at Cadiz Springs

It was unseasonably warm for Wisconsin, and we were home for the Christmas holiday. The kids were still sleeping, except for my daughter who sat in the kitchen having donuts with her Nonnie. It felt peaceful yet absent without the pull, the pressure to walk down the street to my grandparents' or climb the green steps to my parents' house.

Chris rolled over and grabbed my hand. "Why don't we go out and take a look?" he asked.

I hesitated. "I don't have any warm clothes."

All I had packed for this weekend was a Christmas church service outfit, a dress coat, and pajamas.

"Come on, you can borrow my tennis shoes," he said.

And so, I agreed. It wasn't about having the right clothes. I just didn't know if I was ready to head out there and see it yet. Shortly after we sent the check to the Friends of Cadiz Springs State Park, I emailed back and forth with the woman in charge of the non-profit association. I cannot make up these small-town connections, and she remembered me and especially my sister, as she was the youth group leader for a church program where my sister had also found love and acceptance as a teenager. This volunteer was thrilled to work with us on placing a memorial bench along the hiking trail and had recently emailed me to say that the installation was finished.

We bundled up as best we could, got in the car and headed out to Browntown on Highway 11. The familiar turn and path up the winding drive looked different, covered in snow and ice, but it was recognizable all the same. We parked in the lot and got out.

"I'm pretty sure it'll be right down this way," Chris said, always a better navigator than me.

We had asked them to place the bench in view of Beckman Lake, a perfect backdrop to watch raptors soar. We started walking, my feet sloppy in his shoes, and hadn't come too far down the path before we saw it, a bench that looked new, grounded in freshly poured cement. I walked up to it carefully and examined the gold plate on the backrest. My dad's name, birth and death dates were printed on a small placard in the middle, simple and modest.

"Well, take a seat, see how it feels," Chris said, and I sat down.

I took in the view, and it was nice. It was absolutely quiet except for the wind blowing, rustling nearby tree branches and any leaves that were left on them. The water was frozen, but I imagined it lapping against the shore in the warmer months ahead. I pictured people coming here for days to come and sitting on this bench, maybe some people reading the sign and asking, "Who was this guy?" Most people likely not caring, just happy for a place to rest.

"Dad would have loved this view," I said.

"I agree," Chris said.

Infrequent tears slipped slowly down my cheeks. I thought about how different his life, and ours, could have been, if we'd had more science and less shame and secrecy, earlier diagnosis, and community support. But Dad's struggle shaped me into the person I am, and my only lasting regret was that he couldn't see me now.

People say if you see a Cardinal or other special birds, it's a visitor from Heaven with a message for you. I'm not really sure about that. I didn't know if Dad was looking down and watching us, but as I gazed across the ice, I heard a shrill cry in the air. We looked up, and through the clouds the sun peeked through for a minute. A Red-tailed hawk soared across the sky, and with majestic wings outstretched and spanning, he called and swirled.

I blinked, and just like that, it was gone.

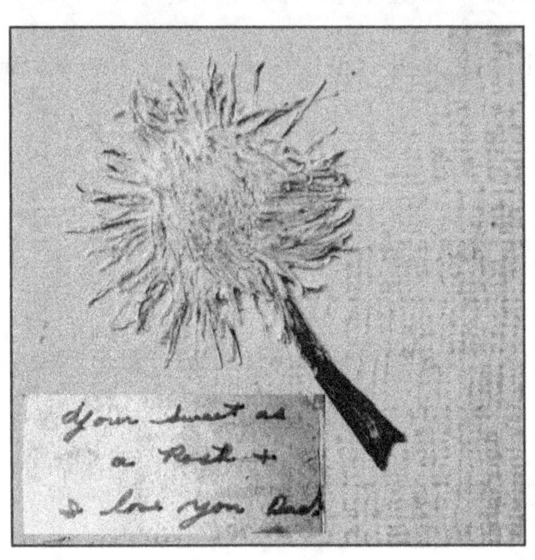

EPILOGUE
Dust Storm

I thought the dust might settle. I was spared from Huntington's disease. My husband and I had hung up our guardian hats and sparked awareness and philanthropy for HD, both in my family and in the local community. But despite my assumption and hope that life would return to normal, I couldn't shake "The Shakes" and found myself in a dark place. For several years after my father died, I felt like I was treading water, and the shoreline was becoming increasingly hard to see.

Where to start? I didn't feel worthy of the HDSA, there were so many affected people who needed help, more than me. My survivor's guilt, while common to many gene-negative individuals, had kept me away from the very support groups who would have understood and accepted me.

From my workplace Employee Assistance Program (EAP) I found a list of resources and a wealth of information and anonymity, for which I was grateful, feeling private and vulnerable about my struggles. The first therapist I chose came from a Christian counseling agency, and her stock advice was to pray more intentionally. She lasted approximately 24 hours.

My next therapist dropped the F-bomb frequently and without remorse, and yet she listened intently, notepad in hand, leaning forward while I introduced myself and my family background during our first session. It was a lot, and after I finished, we sat there quietly.

I asked her weakly, "So, can you fix me?"

She smiled. "We've got some work to do, but I can help you fix yourself."

This one stuck. In weekly sessions, we labored through tough material, using the Cognitive Behavioral Therapy (CBT) method to capture and record thoughts. She validated me and my experiences, saying that, while perception can become a person's reality, I had also actually gone through some shit.

A few months in she asked a question. "Do you think that your father did the best he could with what he had?"

"No way, he could have done so much better," I said, arms folded across my chest.

My dad's illness did not absolve him, and my hurt was

too deep.

We then added eye movement desensitization and reprocessing (EMDR) to my treatment plan. EMDR therapy is a mental health treatment technique which involves moving your eyes while processing traumatic memories. It sounded like Voodoo magic.

First, she explained how it worked. "It doesn't erase your memory. I'm not 'The Men in Black,' and this isn't a 'blinky pen'."

I laughed at her dark humor.

"But it's going to make it less, less..." she paused searching for the word.

"Less of a punch in the gut?" I asked, finishing her sentence with a question.

"Precisely," she answered.

I won't ever discount the power of prayer for the heart, but this formidable therapist brought relief to my brain. After several sessions of EMDR, I could recount difficult memories with reduced physical reactions of fight or flight. No, my dad's illness didn't absolve him of his actions, but it wasn't as simple as that, and we continued to unravel the layers.

If I forgave him, he would still be accountable. Was I ready to set down the load of pain and resentment I had been carrying? With a mash-up of faith and science I came to a place of healing, processed how living with HD in my family has shaped me, and was able to write this book.

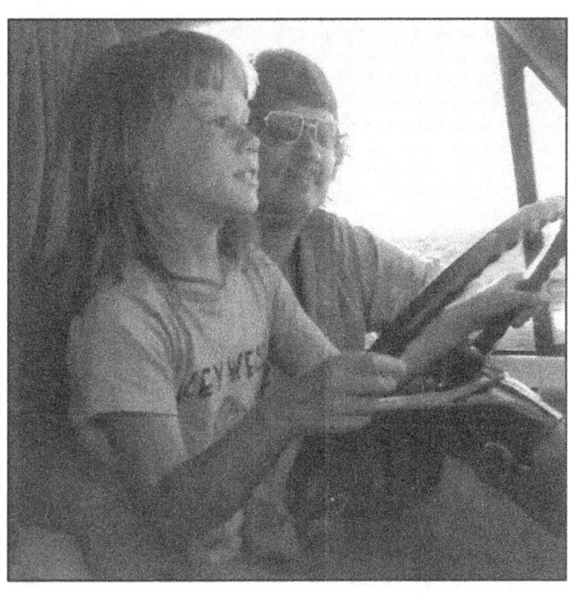

Huntington's disease is a fatal genetic disorder that causes the progressive breakdown of nerve cells in the brain. It deteriorates a person's physical and mental abilities usually during their prime working years and has no cure. Every child of a parent with HD has a 50/50 chance of inheriting the faulty gene that causes the disease. Today, there are approximately 41,000 symptomatic Americans and more than 200,000 at-risk of inheriting the disease. Huntington's disease is described as having ALS, Parkinson's, and Alzheimer's – simultaneously. HD is characterized by a triad of symptoms, including progressive motor dysfunction, behavioral disturbance, and cognitive decline. – HDSA

The Huntington's Disease Society of America (HDSA) is the premier nonprofit organization dedicated to improving the lives of everyone affected by Huntington's disease. From community services and education to advocacy and research, HDSA is the world's leader in providing help for today, hope for tomorrow for people with Huntington's disease and their families. In the battle against Huntington's disease no one fights alone.

https://hdsa.org

ABOUT THE AUTHOR

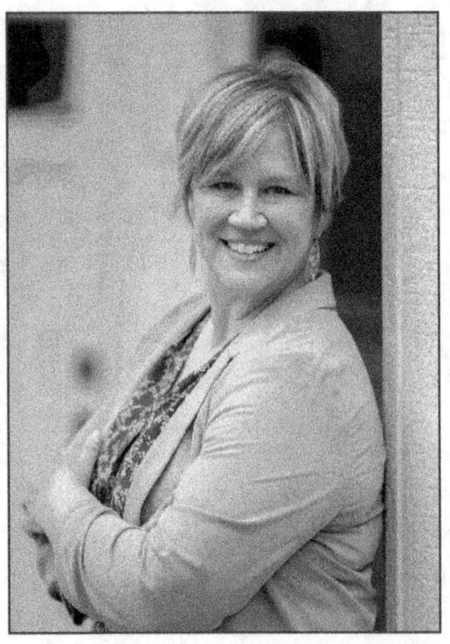

Lori Jones personally experienced the effects of Huntington's Disease (HD) in her family and was instrumental in starting Team Hope Fox Valley events to raise awareness and support for research and community programs through the Huntington's Disease Society of America (HDSA) – Wisconsin Chapter. A storyteller at heart, she regularly writes and speaks about her experiences with HD and many other topics to groups of all ages. Lori has three adult children and lives with her husband Chris in Wisconsin, when they aren't escaping to their cottage in Michigan's Upper Peninsula to enjoy kayaking, hiking, and campfires.

This is her first book.

https://lorijoneswrites.com